TRAUMA

End-of-
Life
Optimum
Support

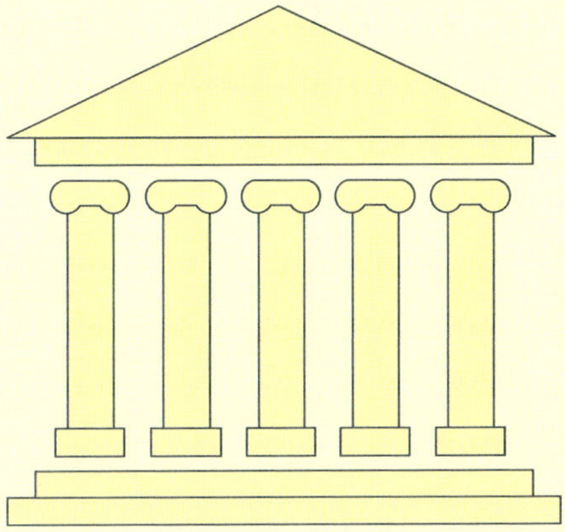

A BEST PRACTICE MODEL
FOR TRAUMA PROFESSIONALS

To Jackie,
Thank you for embracing ethics.
Love, Barbara Jacobs

BARBARA BENNETT JACOBS, PHD, MPH, RN, CHPN

LENWORTH M. JACOBS, MD, MPH, FACS

KARYL BURNS, PHD, RN

Distributed by: Ciné-Med Publishing, Inc.
127 Main Street North
Woodbury, CT 06798

ISBN: 978-0-9824514-4-1

Printed in Canada.

TABLE OF CONTENTS

AUTHORS

Dr. Barbara Bennett Jacobs is the Director of the Ethics Consultation Service at Hartford Hospital in Hartford, Connecticut, and Adjunct Faculty at the University of Connecticut.

Dr. Lenworth M. Jacobs, Jr., is a Professor of Surgery and Professor and Chairman of the Department of Traumatology and Emergency Medicine at the University of Connecticut, and Director of Traumatology and Emergency Medicine at Hartford Hospital.

Dr. Karyl Burns is a Research Scientist with the Department of Traumatology and Emergency Medicine at Hartford Hospital.

ACKNOWLEDGEMENTS

We gratefully acknowledge the Aetna Foundation for its support of the development of TELOS (Trauma End-of-Life Optimum Support), a best practice model for trauma professionals to use to care for trauma victims and their families. It was their vision that health professionals be sensitive to the different cultural norms, practices, and beliefs associated with the dying process. Many individuals assisted with the project. We greatly appreciate those individuals who stopped us in the corridor or stopped by offices to share their insights and hopes for improved quality of end-of-life care for this particular, unique and often vulnerable, patient population.

We are grateful to the American Trauma Society for launching this project by inviting leaders in trauma care and bioethics from across the country to participate in a Trauma Leadership Forum where ideas and suggestions were shared for what ought to be included in a best practice model. We are indebted to Nancy Nurge, APRN, who, while a student at the University of Connecticut's School of Nursing, acted as an assistant to the project and made many contributions, from organizing activities, to entering data from original surveys, to offering critical review of the model. Vijay Jayaraman, MD, helped with the preparation of the TELOS book, scenarios for role play, and the Instructor Manual. His contributions added significantly to their design and aesthetic appeal. In addition, we thank all of the "champions" at Hartford Hospital who enthusiastically supported the development of the project in its early days while offering suggestions from their special disciplines. The Sudden Unexplained Death in Childhood Program also provided us with worthwhile insight. We thank the neuro/trauma intensive care unit nurses and the EMTs and paramedics of the East Hartford Fire Department for being the first TELOS "students" who willingly completed surveys and participated in the pilot educational programs.

INTRODUCTION TO TELOS

Unintentional injuries claimed 121,599 lives in the United States in 2006, with an additional 33,300 dying from suicide, 18,573 dying from assault (homicide), 462 from legal intervention/war, and 5,131 from injury events of undetermined intent.[1] The unintentional injury deaths include those from transport accidents, falls, drowning, exposure, accidental poisonings, and exposure to noxious substances.[1] The total combined trauma deaths (179,065) make trauma the fourth leading cause of death in the United States, preceded by major cardiovascular diseases (which includes cerebrovascular diseases) (823,746), malignant neoplasms (559,888), and a category of "all other diseases" (237,421).[1]

Death due to a traumatic event is typically sudden. Those caring for trauma patients rarely know the victims or their values and preferences for end-of-life care (as with those who complete living wills or die from a terminal illness). The nature of the life-threatening injuries typically requires immediate decision making and intervention. Those persons involved with the victim, e.g., parents, spouses, siblings, children, and friends, are overwhelmed with sudden grief, often guilt, and existential suffering. Although much national attention has been given to improving the care for dying persons and their families through the practices of quality palliative care and by using quality indicators for end-of-life care in the intensive care unit[2], there are still concerns related to how, when, and with whom decisions are made at the end of life due to trauma.[3]

This book is intended to help trauma patients and their families heal and flourish even at a time when death is the expected outcome. We believe that best practices specifically designed for the care of dying trauma victims and their families are special because of the unique population they are designed to serve. We also believe that the actions we as health professionals take need to be grounded not only in a physical-therapeutic approach but also in a prudential-wisdom approach so as to fulfill our obligation to reduce pain and suffering at the end of life. TELOS (Trauma End-of-Life Optimum Support) is a Best Practice Model (BPM) for trauma health professionals to use to care for trauma victims and their families.

TELOS is used here as more than an acronym for Trauma End-of-Life Optimum Support. It is a philosophical stance for the best practices in the model. The ancient Greek word *telos* refers to end or purpose.[4] Teleology is a philosophy that posits that natural events, phenomena, or objects are designed for a purpose or a final cause. The final cause or *telos* of the relationship between trauma health professionals and patients is human flourishing. It is this philosophical grounding in teleology that provides health professionals with their moral authority.[5] Best practices that promote and provide quality end-of-life care are the means to this *telos* in that all practices are aimed at helping dying persons and their families flourish within an environment that is supportive, compassionate, caring, and directed towards the end. It is the moral obligation of health professionals to foster this environment using their skills and knowledge to help someone to flourish even at time of death and dying. Threats to human flourishing such as life-threatening injuries to the actual victims and the subsequent suffering of families make these persons all vulnerable to suffering. It is this suffering that ought to motivate health professionals to use these best practices through their moral agency aimed at "*cultivating the virtues of healthy empathy, sustaining compassion toward others, and joining in solidarity with those in need.*"[6]

Death of a trauma victim may occur either in the prehospital setting, the emergency department, or during the victim's hospital stay in the intensive care unit or non-intensive care settings. Guidelines for TELOS best practices span the categories of:

- Decision making
- Communication
- Spiritual care
- Culturally-sensitive social care
- Psychological care

The majority of the best practices reflect a specific practice for decision making, communication, spiritual care, and culturally-sensitive social care. However, practices related to psychological care are embedded in the other categories because it is our belief that attention to the psychological responses to the injury event by the patient and the family should not be isolated, but rather integrated into all practices. The practices are designed to be implemented with a firm foundation in engagement, ethics, education, evaluation, and economics.

Words that are **bolded** the first time they appear
in the following pages can be found in the Glossary.
Underlining of certain words is used for emphasis.
Certain key practices are highlighted in yellow.

THE BEST PRACTICE MODEL

The BPM includes a book as well as an Instructor Manual. The book is presented in two sections:

SECTION ONE includes general best practices founded on values and principles associated with what are referred to as pillars. These are *(see Figure 1)*:

- **Engagement** – mutual indebtedness and relationship between patients and health professionals that has, as an end, human flourishing and healing, even at time of death;
- **Ethics** – ethical **comportment** and **moral agency** needed to respond to the ethical issues that arise in clinical practice;
- **Education** – knowledge and skills to be competent to practice best practices in the areas of physical, psychological, emotional, social, religious/spiritual, and cultural domains;
- **Evaluation** – process needed to ensure the development, implementation, testing, and monitoring of the BPM; and
- **Economics** – financial and administrative support for the stability and sustainability of the BPM over time.

SECTION TWO includes specific best practices for implementation in three settings:

- PREHOSPITAL SETTING
- EMERGENCY DEPARTMENT
- INTENSIVE CARE UNIT

SECTION TWO also includes the following:

- REFERENCES
- GLOSSARY
- APPENDICES

THE INSTRUCTOR MANUAL contains educational materials divided into three sections, one section for the education of prehospital professionals, the second section for education of emergency department professionals, and the third section for education of intensive care unit professionals. Each section contains: 1) Sample Applications for Continuing Education Credit, 2) Confidence Assessment Instrument, 3) Frequency Assessment Instrument, 4) Knowledge Assessment Instrument, 5) Presentation Materials, and 6) Scenarios to Use for Role-play or Boalean Theater.[7–8] The scenarios are also in Appendix 1 of the **TELOS** book. The Confidence Assessment measures *how confident* respondents are performing certain best practices, the Frequency Assessment measures *how often* respondents perform certain best practices, and the Knowledge Assessment asks multiple choice questions related to the subject material contained in the best practices. All three instruments can be used to perform a needs assessment prior to organizing a TELOS program, as well as be administered prior to and after a program for evaluation purposes.

The scripted scenarios may be used for conventional role-play and are also conducive to **Boalean Theater Forum**.[7,8] Boalean Theater Forum is an adaptation of theater developed by Augusto Boal who founded the Theater of the Oppressed. The actors (health professionals acting *qua* health professional or *qua* patient or family) perform a play with a script. At any point during the play, any "spect-actor" from the audience attending the educational program may clap his/her hands and call out "stop!" and then take the place of the actor portraying any one individual already on the stage. In other words, those in the audience listening to the script are not just idle spectators (audience) but can participate in the action on stage as "spect-actors."

As Boal stated:

> *Communication between actor and audience takes place at two levels: 'wave' and 'underwave' or 'undercurrent.' Actors communicate to an audience on a conscious level, by means of the thoughts they 'emit.' When an actor's thoughts are not in accord with his action – i.e., when there is a clash between wave and undercurrent – the audience/receiver experiences a phenomenon similar to interference on the radio; the audience receives two contradictory messages and it is impossible to register them both.*[7]

The objective of this technique is to respect the "other's" view of how to approach a particular situation using, in this case, TELOS best practices. An additional objective is to recognize and respect the voices of the many "players" involved in difficult situations that arise at the end of life. Emory University has used a similar technique called "Readers Theater"[9] and Yale University has used role-play to incorporate training in spirituality into medical education.[10]

CAVEAT ONE

Any practice outlined in this BPM that is in opposition to laws, regulations, policies, protocols, guidelines, or procedures of another state or institution should not be followed until such opposition can be resolved. Connecticut guidelines and public health codes are provided only as examples. Users of this book need to be aware of examples for their own states.

CAVEAT TWO

TELOS, by design and intention, does not address best practices for the physical care of patients, (medical, nursing, or prehospital clinical management of trauma victims). Numerous courses, textbooks, and guidelines are available for the physical management of compromises to the anatomical and physiological integrity of trauma victims.

- For surgical clinical management by physicians, see the Advanced Trauma Operative Management (ATOM) course.
  Access at: www.harthosp.org/ATOM
- For clinical management by physicians, see the Advanced Trauma Life Support Course offered by the American College of Surgeons.
  Access at: http://www.facs.org/trauma/atls/index.html
- For clinical management by nurses, see the Trauma Nurse Core Course (TNCC) and the Course in Advanced Trauma Nursing (CATN) offered by the Emergency Nurses Association.
  Access at: http://www.ena.org/catn_enpc_tncc/tncc/
- Advanced Trauma Care for Nurses (ATCN) offered by the Society for Trauma Nurses. Access at: http://www.traumanurses.org/atch-courses.html
- For clinical management by prehospital personnel, see the Prehospital Trauma Life Support Course offered by the National Association of EMTs.
  Access at: http://www.naemt.org/PHTLS/aboutPHTLS/

FIGURE 1

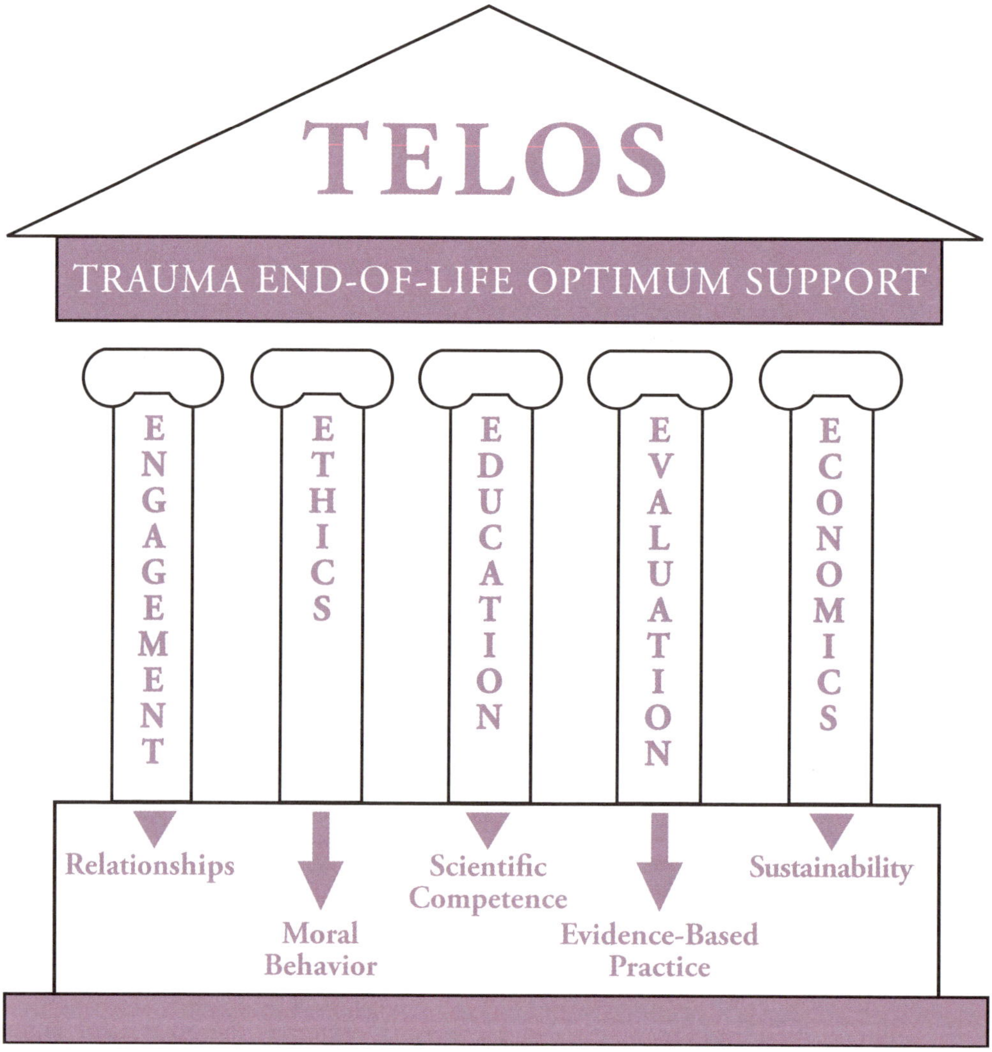
TELOS
TRAUMA END-OF-LIFE OPTIMUM SUPPORT
ENGAGEMENT
ETHICS
EDUCATION
EVALUATION
ECONOMICS
Relationships
Moral Behavior
Scientific Competence
Evidence-Based Practice
Sustainability

INTRODUCTION TO GENERAL PRACTICES RELATED TO THE FIVE PILLARS

The following five sections include general best practices related to the pillars of the TELOS BPM in the specific categories of engagement, ethics, education, evaluation, and economics. These practices are intended for implementation with those practices specific to each of the following environments: prehospital, emergency department, or intensive care unit.

The goal of trauma care is to save patients' lives and restore persons to their preinjury health status. However, there is significant mortality associated with trauma. Some victims die instantly and are never transported to a hospital. Others are so critically injured that their death may occur en route, shortly after arrival in the emergency department, operating room, or intensive care unit or after a prolonged hospitalization. All victims need expert clinical management and stabilization of their injuries. Families and significant other persons important to the patient also require the attention and care of health professionals involved in the patient's care. An integrated plan of palliative care oriented to pain and symptom management and compassionate caring at the end of life may be the desired goal for those patients whose survival is unlikely.

Transporting patients with no likelihood of survival to trauma centers and implementing aggressive resuscitation efforts are often empirically and morally questionable and consume valuable human and financial resources. For hospitalized patients and families, the failure to recognize that aggressive care is no longer effective and that a focus on **palliative care** is a better option may have negative consequences. The painful prolongation of dying and the overuse of critical resources may limit the ability to address clinical, emotional, spiritual, and psychological issues in a meaningful manner. The decision to transition the focus from aggressive, injury-specific care to palliative care is a decision often fraught with uncertainty, lack of consensus between the medical team and family, and poor timing.

The purpose of this BPM is to provide health professionals with practices that promote quality end-of-life care specifically for trauma victims and their families. The TELOS BPM is a synthesis of recommendations from:

1. Two trauma leadership forums sponsored by the American Trauma Society where experts in the field of trauma gathered and made recommendations for a BPM.

2. A public survey of 1,006 persons that garnered the public's attitudes and beliefs related to, for example, family presence during resuscitation, importance of comfort, **advanced care planning**, organ donation, life in a **persistent vegetative state (PVS)**, importance of religion and spiritual beliefs, and cultural sensitivity.[11]

3. A professional survey of 774 EMS providers, physicians, nurses, social workers, and chaplains related to the same issues cited above.[11] Both the public survey and the professional survey were conducted by the authors of TELOS to discover important beliefs of the public and professionals so as to provide documented evidence-based research to support the best practices.

4. Review of the literature.

ENGAGEMENT PRACTICES

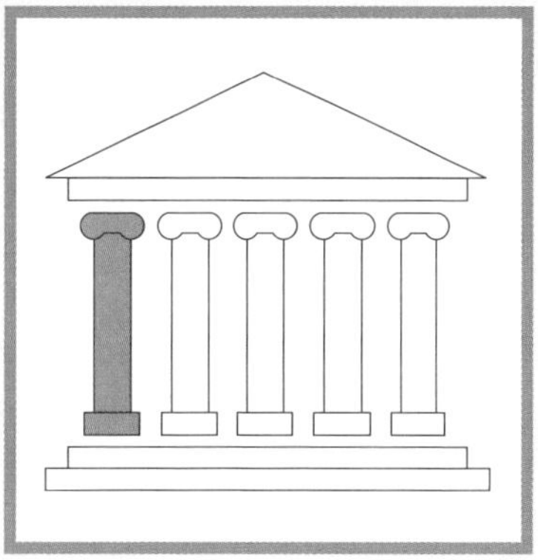

Engagement refers to the mutual indebtedness between patients and health professionals. Ethical engagement goes beyond objective or subjective certainty into a realm of **intersubjective contingency** where the relationship between a patient and a health professional is one of respect for the **existential** nature of those persons involved (the uniqueness of each other).[12] This postmodern view of the health professional/patient relationship as a covenant contributes to the stability and sustainability of the model over time. The engagement between patients and health professionals spans the physical, psychological, emotional, social, religious, spiritual, and cultural domains of care. Assessment of, and interventions for the well-being or **human flourishing** of the patient, engages all the stakeholders in order to develop and implement a plan of care that is based in a philosophy of the **ethics of care** through engagement that is authentic and patient-centered.

Engagement with society as a whole for establishing societal values as related to end-of-life care is ongoing and ought to be supported by members of the trauma team. Encouraging such dialogue through open forums specific to morally challenging concerns that end of life brings forth, e.g., brain death, prolonging life in a vegetative state through life-sustaining treatments, organ donation incentive programs, or admission criteria, heightens the public's attention to these issues. Public dialogue can provide a moral space for such reflection. Care in the psychological domain is integrated into the following engagement-related practices. The following practices are specific to the model's foundation in engagement.

ENGAGEMENT: GENERAL PRACTICES

Engagement 1

Relate to the patient and or his/her **surrogate** decision maker through an engagement of care that grounds the relationship in the recognition that each patient is unique with a life narrative (story) that is meaningful and interpreted by the patient and/or family.

Engagement 2

Establish a **fiduciary (trust) relationship** between health professionals and patients of all ages, **races**, **ethnicities**, religions, and spiritual beliefs.

Engagement 3

Recognize that the majority of the public trust health professionals and then build the new relationship of engagement on that foundation of trust.[11]

Engagement 4

Function as a member of the **interprofessional team** to communicate with other team members, to provide patients and families consistent and accurate information, and to resolve conflicts or problems through consensus and collaboration when formulating or revising a patient's plan of care.

ENGAGEMENT: COMMUNICATION PRACTICES

Engagement 5

Converse with patients and/or their family members specifically attuned to:

5.1 their style of engagement, e.g., some families may prefer to start a conversation about end-of-life issues with a prayer, others may prefer to hear first from the physician in charge, others may need an interpreter or prefer to have a family member who is familiar with medical language be involved

5.2 the uniqueness of each family and each family member; avoid stereotyping based on age, race, gender, or ethnicity

5.3 your style of engagement that may need to be modified based on the responses of the patient and family members

5.4 the appropriate language level of individual family members according to age, developmental and comprehension level

Engagement 6

Demonstrate <u>professionalism</u> (in voice and overall appearance), competency, confidence, and avoid appearing rushed, arrogant or hostile.

6.1 Devote your attention to these conversations; suggest to other staff that you not be disturbed during these conversations.

Engagement 7

Establish a **<u>communicative rapport</u>** when having conversations with family members.

7.1 Arrange a comfortable location for families to wait, e.g., couches to rest on, access to food and fluids, availability of a telephone, privacy, access to rest rooms, and aesthetically appropriate decor.[13]

7.2 Introduce yourself and your role in the healthcare team.

7.3 Be aware of the patient's name and use that name when communicating with the family.[13]

7.4 Learn the relationships to the patient of the family members to whom you are engaging in conversation.

7.5 Position yourself close to the patient's closest relative, spouse, or significant other person—sit if possible, and look the relative directly in his/her eyes when speaking; make a judgment as to whether touching would be perceived as appropriate.[13]

7.6 Display **empathy**, which is the understanding of another's thoughts and feelings and communicating that understanding to them.[14]

7.7 Correct any misconceptions or misinterpretations of information.

7.8 Listen to the response of the patient and/or family members and be prepared to give time for reactions of fear, guilt, hostility, anger, denial, and even a cathartic response of nonacceptance.

7.9 Determine, if possible, what positive coping skills relatives may have used in the past and encourage their use now.

7.10 Identify those persons relatives may want contacted for social support.

7.11 Recognize that periods of silence may help families process information.

7.12 Encourage relatives to express their feelings and do not discourage crying.

Engagement 8

Engage in **caring communication** that demonstrates compassion, sensitivity, consistency, truthfulness, and is timely.

8.1 Respect the ethical principle of **veracity** and avoid deceit.

8.2 Respond to the reaction of patients and families that such communication may precipitate.

8.3 Avoid labeling a family as difficult. Such labeling jeopardizes the fiduciary relationship between patients and healthcare team members.

Engagement 9

Engage in conversations with families to relate poor prognosis, imminent death, or actual death, while following *Engagement 5-8*.

9.1 The most senior physician should provide the above communication. Avoid passing off this engagement practice (and responsibility) to junior resident physicians.

9.2 Avoid phrases like *"meaningful recovery"* or words that have vague interpretations which families may have problems defining.

9.3 Avoid euphemisms, e.g., *"passed on"*

9.4 Foster consistency in the use of certain words by members of the health care team, e.g., *"died"* instead of *"expired."* However, attempt to learn from families what words may upset them; some persons find the harshness of the word "*died*" too overwhelming.

9.5 Do not say, *"I know how you feel"*; some persons may perceive this phrase as offensive since one does not really know how another feels. It also may shut down the conversation.

9.6 Relieve family's worry that their loved one is suffering or may have suffered.

9.6.1 Inform the family that the patient did not feel pain or suffer especially if the patient was unresponsive or dead on arrival.

9.6.2 If the patient is alive and complaining of pain, inform the family that appropriate medication will be given to relieve the pain.

Engagement 10

Discuss a traumatic event or death of a loved one with a child based on the child's developmental level.

10.1 Determine if the parent of the child is available and in a psychological state that permits reasonable communication to tell the child of a traumatic event or a death.

10.1.1 If not, attempt to locate another family member to discuss and decide who should inform the child.

10.2 A designated trauma team representative should accompany the parent or other family member to be supportive and answer questions.

10.3 Determine the child's perception of death.

10.4 Be specific and avoid euphemisms, as children may interpret them literally.

10.5 Avoid platitudes that children may not understand, e.g., *"time will heal your grief."*

10.6 Use silence and patience for the news to be processed by the child.

10.7 Reinforce that the death was not preventable and all that could be done to save the patient was done, that the child was not responsible for the event or death, and that to cry and feel very sad is appropriate.

10.8 Evaluate the child's reaction to the news and respond appropriately. A child may feel guilty, abandoned, and rejected.

10.9 Involve a child development specialist as time permits.

ENGAGEMENT: DECISION-MAKING PRACTICES

Engagement 11

Engage in care of the patient based on the established goal of care determined through **shared decision making** ***with the patient and/or the patient's valid surrogate and the interprofessional team.***

11.1 Three **types of care** are as follows:

11.1.1 aggressive curative care that is injury- or disease- specific

11.1.2 life-sustaining medical care, e.g., mechanical ventilation, artificial hydration and nutrition, cardiopulmonary resuscitation (CPR)

11.1.3 ***Palliative comfort care is a type of care that is always provided, whether or not it is the specific focus with or without injury-specific curative care and/or life-sustaining medical care.***

11.2 It is the emphasis on a particular type of care that requires discussion with appropriate surrogates and those healthcare team members responsible for the patient's care.[15]

11.3 Help families transition from emphasis on one type of care, e.g., aggressive, to focus on another type of care, e.g., palliative only.

11.3.1 Reinforce that palliative care is always provided within all three types of care.

11.3.2 ***Correct any misperception that a patient will not receive expert, attentive care when the focus is palliation.***

11.3.3 Answer consistently and accurately all questions that families may have related to types of care or goals of care.

11.3.4 Frequently discuss the type of care the patient is receiving with families.

Engagement 12

Recognize and respond to threats to engagement.

12.1 Obtain legal opinion if there are discrepancies as to who is the authorized, legally valid surrogate in the event that the patient does not have the **decision-making capacity** to make his/her healthcare decisions.

12.2 Use a shared decision-making method when there is a lack of consensus as to the appropriate goals of care, e.g., consensus between individual family members, consensus between family members and health care team, consensus between healthcare team members.

12.3 ***Consult with the Ethics Committee or Ethics Consultation Service when there is a stalemate in consensus-driven, shared decision-making.***

12.4 Consult with Social Services or Pastoral Care Services when conflicts arise.

12.5 Utilize other best practices including *Engagement 7-9*, *Ethics 9-12 and 19-22*, and *Intensive Care Unit 10-23*.

ENGAGEMENT: CULTURAL PRACTICES

Engagement 13

Assess the patient and the family from a cultural perspective in order to integrate cultural awareness and diversity into a plan for culturally sensitive and culturally competent care. Include answers to questions and information from the following domains[16]:

13.1 Heritage – origin, residence, education, occupation

13.2 Communication – language, use of dialects, eye contact, greetings, touch, names, spatial distancing, volume/tone of voice, facial expressions

13.3 Family roles and organization – head of household, gender roles, goals and priorities, roles of elders, extended family, social status, alternative lifestyle, developmental tasks

13.4 Nutrition – meaning of food, common foods, rituals, limitations

13.5 Death rituals – praying and other religious rituals or sacraments, chanting, anointing oils, who can touch the body

13.6 Spirituality – religion, religious practices, use of prayer, meaning of life and death, belief in miracles and Divine Intervention

13.7 Health care practices – traditions, customs, pain and sick role responses

Engagement 14

Use carefully general information about certain groups that can be found in guide books that list certain characteristics of specific cultural groups[16], as needed.

14.1 Avoid artificially stereotyping individuals as this may jeopardize your relationship.

14.2 Remember that variation among individuals of the same **culture** is possible since everyone does not adhere to the same intracultural norms.[17-18]

Engagement 15

Recognize and respect that individuals of the same culture may demonstrate cultural variation and the broad stereotypical beliefs about a certain culture may not help to predict a response.[17-18]

ENGAGEMENT: SPIRITUAL/RELIGIOUS PRACTICES

Engagement 16

Identify and respect the **spiritual concerns** and/or religious beliefs of patients and their families.

16.1 A spiritual history may be obtained using the suggested acronym FICA: F for faith and beliefs, I for importance of spirituality in the lives of the patients and the family, C for the community of support the patient/family may use, A for how the patient/family wishes spiritual issues to be addressed.[19]

16.2 A spiritual history may be obtained using the suggested acronym SPIRIT: S for the spiritual belief system, P for personal spirituality, I for integration within a spiritual community, R for rituals (practices and restrictions), I for implications of spiritual beliefs on medical care, and T for terminal events planning.[19]

Engagement 17

Recognize a patient's or family's religious or spiritual belief that Divine Intervention is possible.

17.1 Obtain an ethics consult or pastoral care consult if the family's belief in Divine Intervention (e.g., miracle) is stalemating a discussion of realistic goals of care.

Engagement 18

Assess for needs of the patient and/or family as related to spiritual/religious care.

18.1 Intervene to meet the above needs, e.g., pastoral care consult, contact of specifically requested spiritual or religious church leader.

18.2 Respond to a request for prayer by praying with the patient or contacting a member of the Pastoral Care Team.

Engagement 19

Avoid reframing a patient's religious or spiritual perspectives.

Engagement 20

Recognize signs of positive religious coping, e.g., *"I look to God for strength, support, and guidance,"* as well as signs of negative religious coping, e.g., *"Why has God abandoned me?"*[19]

Engagement 21

Clarify any vague statements about spirituality before overinterpreting.

Engagement 22

Implement spiritual care to meet the specific religious needs of patients who consider such care as important as the patient's physical care.

22.1 ***Medical procedures and treatment can proceed regardless of interruption for spiritual care; do not limit access of pastoral care representatives into the room of a dying patient.***

22.2 Recognize the importance of traditional religious beliefs of the dying, e.g., Catholicism and the Annointing of the Sick, Islamic belief in facing Mecca and being surrounded by loved ones, Hinduism and the strong preference to die at home, and the importance of chanting.

Engagement 23

Obtain a pastoral care consult.

Engagement 24

Share any assessment of the patient's and/or family's spiritual/religious needs and plans for intervention with the interprofessional team.

ENGAGEMENT: DEATH AND DYING PRACTICES

Engagement 25

Engage patients and their families in relationships that are sensitive to their reactions and responses to the trauma event, the dying process, and the event of death.

25.1 ***Determine availability of any verbal or written advance directives while conveying the urgency to do so in a calm, solicitous way.***

25.2 Assess emotional responses and support with interventions that reduce existential and physical suffering.

25.3 Assess spiritual responses and support with interventions that respect these responses and reduce suffering.

25.4 Provide access to persons who represent the religious and/or cultural preferences of the patient and family, as requested.

25.5 Refer families to bereavement services or counseling and follow-up to ensure that their needs for such services are being addressed.

25.6 Design a bereavement plan for follow-up that can be implemented and revised as needed.

Engagement 26

Assess whether family members may find comfort from a remembrance of their loved one in the event of death, e.g., handprint, footprint of a child, or a lock of hair, and then offer to procure such a remembrance and provide an aesthetically comforting package for its transport.

26.1 Prepare personal belongings and effects to give to family members in such a way that minimizes a traumatic response.

ENGAGEMENT: INTERPROFESSIONAL HEALTHCARE TEAM ENGAGEMENT PRACTICES

Engagement 27

Support healthcare team members from all environments through programs, support services, stress-debriefing sessions, or individual counseling sessions designed to meet their needs for psychological adjustment to stressful and disturbing circumstances associated with caring for patients at the end of life.

27.1 Consider providing relief from the workplace to a healthcare professional who is too distressed to continue work after a particularly disturbing incident.

27.2 Sessions should be voluntary, and not mandated in order to meet individual needs unless there is some specific reason that all professionals involved in a particular incident are required to attend, e.g., review of a system design issue.

ENGAGEMENT: COMMUNITY PRACTICES

Engagement 28

Consider engaging in societal dialogues related to end-of-life issues yourself with other members of a community (local, statewide, or national) to provide a space for all persons to have a moral voice free of constraints.

28.1 Consider becoming involved in discussions with local church groups, book clubs, and professional organizations *(see Appendix 2: Suggested Topics for Public Discourse and Dialogue)*.

28.2 Consider becoming involved with statewide groups such as EMS councils, advisory boards to health agencies and organizations, and public health work groups.

28.3 Consider becoming involved in national professional groups or national organizations like the American Trauma Society and Mothers Against Drunk Driving.

ETHICS PRACTICES

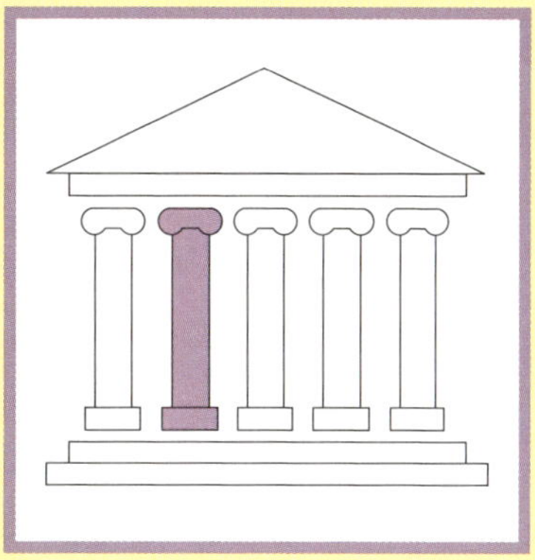

The moral imperative of health professionals is reflected in ethical comportment and moral agency.[20] It encompasses how to recognize and respond to moral challenges, to reason and formulate options in the best interest of the patient, and to justify options through shared decision making with patients and their healthcare decision makers. Professional ethics reinforces the stability and sustainability of the BPM over time. Ethical competence has significance in the physical, psychological, emotional, social, religious, spiritual, and cultural domains of patient care. Assessment of these domains of well-being or human flourishing of persons is essential in order to develop and implement a plan of care that is ethically sound, authentic and patient-centered. Care in the psychological domain is integrated into the following ethics-related practices. The following practices are specific to the model's foundation in ethics.

ETHICS: GENERAL PRACTICES

Ethics 1

***Answer the therapeutic and* prudential question*—
What are the right (based on scientific and empirical evidence), and good actions (based on patient's values and preferences) that are in the best interest of the patient?*[21]**

Ethics 2

Respect and honor the personal **autonomy** of all patients and those surrogates who are representing the patient's values and beliefs for treatment whether verbally or through written living wills.

Ethics 3

Recognize the value and worth of patients from the time of the injury event through death by respecting their intrinsic ***dignity*** *as humans and attributing dignity to them.*

3.1 To respect someone's intrinsic dignity is to respect the moral personhood of human beings because they have the potential to make their own choices about their own lives. Intrinsic dignity can never be *"lost"* and no one dies *"without dignity."*

3.2 Dignity that is considered attributed dignity is the dignity others attribute, show, or demonstrate to another person or the dignity a person attributes to him/herself. Such dignity attribution can change over time depending on the person's circumstances. Injury or death can *"attack"* the dignity one attributes to him/herself by *"robbing"* one of control and independence.[22]

3.3 ***All patients have moral standing based on the criteria that they have the capacity for pain, suffering, and emotional deprivation.[23] These criteria are the moral basis for attributing dignity and respect to those human beings who cannot express themselves.***

Ethics 4

Respect the age, race, ethnicity, cultural heritage, and religion of all patients. Discrimination of any kind in any form, e.g., against patients with certain pre-existing medical disorders, age, disabilities, or social status, must never occur and if it does, ought to carry significant reprimand.

Ethics 5

Treat all patients equally on a timely basis; avoid preferential care based on social or political status.

Ethics 6

Identify the values, beliefs, preferences, and advance directives (living will, healthcare representative designation) of patients and their surrogates that may influence their decision making. Such identification includes an assessment of spiritual beliefs, cultural values, and a general psychosocial evaluation.

Ethics 7

Respect the patient's and family's **privacy**; that by its very nature protects the patient from any unauthorized intrusion.

7.1 Allow only those persons responsible for the patient's care to have access to patient information, e.g., written and computerized protected health information (PHI).

7.2 Do not discuss patients with anyone who does not have the legal and/or moral authority to be involved in the patient's care.

7.3 Follow hospital procedures for privacy practices related to PHI.

Ethics 8

Respect the patient's and family's **confidentiality** by protecting private health information and do not disclose such information without the patient's **consent**.[24]

Ethics 9

Utilize a shared decision-making model to determine the goals of care that respect the patient's (and/or surrogate's) values and beliefs, but do not compromise the professional integrity of health professionals.[21]

Ethics 10

Employ an interprofessional team whose members accept responsibility to cooperate to achieve the *"good"* for each patient by adhering to the TELOS BPM.

Ethics 11

Formulate a plan and interventions using the interprofessional team to assess and manage symptoms causing physical pain and suffering.

Ethics 12

Formulate a plan and interventions using the interprofessional team to assess and manage existential symptoms (nonphysical) that are causing pain and suffering, e.g., patient's concern of the value and meaning of life.

Ethics 13

*Nurture a professional moral character or moral agency that represents the **virtues of health professionals**, e.g., **fidelity** to trust and promise, benevolence, effacement of self-interest, compassion, caring, intellectual honesty, **justice**, prudence or practical wisdom.[25]*

Ethics 14

Respond to challenges (i.e., situations that may cause you to question your involvement in particular actions) to your moral agency and professional integrity in such a way that your response does not jeopardize care to the patient and/or family or place them at risk for further injury.

14.1 Do not **abandon** a patient to avoid participating in an action that challenges moral or professional integrity.

14.1.1 Identify another health professional to assume patient care in the event that you perceive your continued involvement is a violation of your moral or professional integrity.

14.1.2 Establish plans in advance to respond to individual challenges to moral and professional integrity.

14.1.3 Require supervisory support for health professionals who decide to opt out of care that is against their personal beliefs and values as a health professional.

14.1.4 Use advocacy and leadership skills to bring attention to situations that lead to moral distress[26] before such moral distress compromises integrity resulting in moral residue ("*that which each of us carries with us from those times in our lives when in the face of moral distress we have seriously compromised ourselves or allowed ourselves to be compromised.*")[26]

14.1.5 Request an ethics consult, as needed.

Ethics 15

Perform cardiopulmonary resuscitation according to the American Heart Association's guidelines as indicated. Slow coding, chemical coding, or any practice that is not according to the standards is unacceptable and is considered deceit even though the intention is to be nonmaleficent or not intended to cause harm.

ETHICS: CONSENT/REFUSAL PRACTICES

Ethics 16

Obtain consent or refusal for any medical treatment or intervention that requires such consent or refusal, mindful of four essential principles:

16.1 Disclose the following elements of the intervention: nature, purpose, risks and consequences, benefits, probability of success, feasible alternatives, and prognosis with or without the intervention.

16.2 ***Determine decision-making capacity based on the following: patient's ability to understand information necessary to make any one decision at any one point in time, ability to reason in accord with a relatively consistent set of values, ability to communicate preferences.***

16.3 Ask patients or surrogates to repeat in their words what they either consented to or refused to determine comprehension.

16.4 Ensure the patient's or a surrogate's voluntary decision in that it was not manipulated through persuasion or coercion.

Ethics 17

Facilitate the consent/refusal decision process by:

17.1 Identifying the appropriate and legally valid surrogate in the event the patient does not demonstrate adequate decisional capacity.

17.2 Sitting face-to-face with patient or surrogate in a private place without distraction.

17.3 Offering a recommendation.

17.4 Acknowledging and responding to any emotional reaction.

17.5 Validating decision at the end of the conversation.

17.6 Summarizing the discussion, asking questions, and making plans to discuss the treatment or procedure another time if the patient or family requests to do so.

Ethics 18

Evaluate the capacity of those persons younger than18 years of age to participate in treatment decision making (**assent**) along with their parents, by considering the following:

18.1 the awareness the patient has of the nature of his/her condition based on his/her developmental level

18.2 whether the minor has an opinion about his/her willingness to agree to the care or treatment being considered

18.3 document whether the minor agrees with his/her parents' decision

18.4 discuss conflicts with the minor patient and family when the minor's wishes differ from those of the parent or legally valid surrogate

ETHICS: RESOLVING CONFLICTS OF FUTILITY PRACTICES

Ethics 19

Identify, analyze, and attempt to resolve the ethical problems that arise in practice.[27]

Ethics 20

Utilize an ethics consultant or Ethics Committee when ethical conflicts cannot be resolved.

Ethics 21

Consider the two distinctions of medical **futility** before making a futility determination.

21.1 Quantitative futility is the <u>fact distinction</u> – the facts that lead the <u>physician</u> to the determination of physiologic futility, based on scientific and empirical evidence that a certain treatment or intervention will not achieve its biomedical goal or will not alter the natural course of the patient's injuries, or just makes no clinical sense and therefore is not indicated.[28]

21.2 Qualitative futility is the <u>value distinction</u> – values that lead the <u>patient</u> or surrogate to conclude that the treatment has no benefit according to such values.[28]

Ethics 22

Determine medical futility of a treatment by balancing effectiveness, benefits, and burdens, considering that[29]*:*

22.1 Effectiveness of a treatment is an objective determination made by the physician as to whether the treatment in question will be physiologically effective in achieving its intended effect and altering the patient's overall anticipated course.

22.2 Benefits of a treatment are the subjective determination of the patient and/or the patient's decision maker as to the value and desirability of the treatment.

22.3 Burdens are the subjective determinations of the patient and/or surrogate decision maker and the objective determinations of the physician related to, but not limited to cost, comfort, discomfort, pain, quality-of-life assessments.

22.3.1 Burdens related to facts can typically be determined by the physician.

22.3.2 Burdens related to subjective and personal issues of the patient typically can be determined by the patient, family, or surrogate who is representing the patient's values.

22.4 There are reasons that patients and/or their surrogates may request treatments, which in the view of the healthcare team are futile, such as:

22.4.1 religious or spiritual convictions that Divine Intervention will occur[30]

22.4.2 faulty reasoning[30]

22.4.3 unrealistic expectations of survival[30]

22.4.4 inability to trust professional judgment[30]

22.4.5 entitlement or a right-based belief that any treatment ought to be offered[30]

22.4.6 young age of trauma victim and suddenness of death and dying

22.5 Any one particular diagnosis, e.g., gunshot wound to the head, does not indicate that any one subsequent treatment is futile.

ETHICS: JUSTICE PRACTICES

Ethics 23

Be fair and just in all exchanges with patients as individuals while giving to them what is owed in terms of the agreement/relationship between them, their individual health providers, organizations, i.e., hospital (commutative justice).[4]

23.1 Follow the mission of the institution/agency where you are employed.

23.2 Adhere to the values articulated by the institution/agency, e.g., respect, integrity, service, stewardship.

Ethics 24

Allocate and utilize scarce resources based on a fair and equitable plan (distributive justice).[4]

24.1 Follow the organ procurement plan of your local Organ Procurement Organization (OPO) for allocation of organs.

24.2 Adhere to any laws pertaining to the rights of individuals to declare themselves organ donors.

24.3 Adhere to any laws pertaining to the distribution of resources during a public health emergency that may require allocation of scarce resources during a multi-casualty incident resulting in a surge in the number of trauma patients that may exceed capacity.

EDUCATION PRACTICES

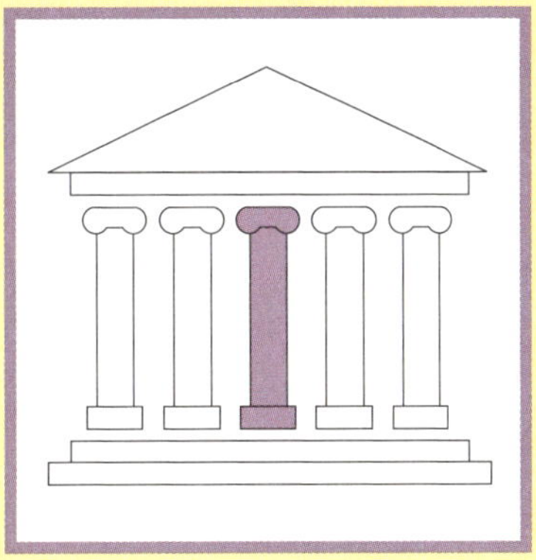

Continuing education to refine and adapt practices cited in the TELOS BPM is essential to the stability and sustainability of the model over time. Education is essential in the areas of physical, psychological, emotional, social, religious, spiritual, and cultural domains of the patient's and family's responses to the injury event. Education of health professionals in the assessment of and interventions for the well-being or human flourishing of persons is tantamount to develop and implement a plan of care that is educationally sound, authentic, and patient-centered.
The following practices are specific to the model's foundation in education.

EDUCATION PRACTICES

Education 1

Develop continuing education and in-service programs specific to each health professional practicing in the three environments, i.e., prehospital, emergency department, or intensive care unit.

Education 2

Implement continuing education and in-service programs specific to the interprofessional team as a unit of learners, e.g., prehospital personnel, physicians, nurses, social workers, pastoral care representatives, mental health professionals.

Education 3

Utilize philosophy of adult learning in all educational programs:

3.1 Foster and reward critical thinking.

3.2 Involve professionals in their own learning.

3.3 Focus on the process of learning as well as the content to be learned.

3.4 Involve professionals in the design of the learning initiatives.

3.5 ***Recognize the value of professionals' previous experiences and its contribution to their learning.***

3.6 Involve professionals in the evaluation of their learning.

3.7 Evaluate feedback from learners and incorporate appropriate suggestions.

Education 4

Incorporate palliative care practice as a core competency into the educational programs.

Education 5

Offer through role-play or simulations, communicating with patients and their families about topics such as: imminent or actual death of a family member, poor prognoses, complicated medical situations, conflict resolution, complex family structures and dynamics, or expectation of death or expectation of recovery.

Education 6

Consider accessing the Education in Palliative and End-of-Life Care (**EPEC**) program via online learning or conference learning. Areas of the EPEC curriculum include: gaps in end-of-life care, legal issues related to palliative care, elements and models of palliative care, pain management, communicating bad news, advance care planning, physician-assisted suicide/euthanasia, whole patient assessment, negotiating goals of care, managing sudden, critical illness, medical futility, conflict resolution, withholding/withdrawing therapy, common physical symptoms, depression, anxiety, delirium, last hours of living.[31]

Education 7

Consider accessing the educational program offered through The End-of-Life Nursing Education Consortium (**ELNEC**) project of the Association of the American Colleges of Nursing (AACN).[32]

Education 8

Consider modeling a TELOS educational program in your facility using this BPM.

EVALUATION PRACTICES

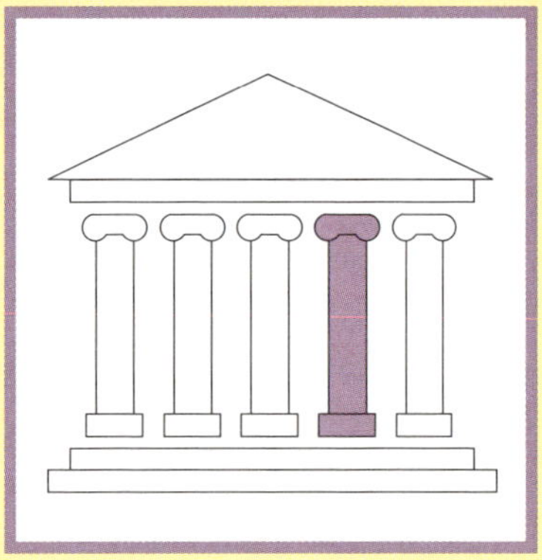

Evaluation is the process needed to ensure that the development, implementation, testing, and monitoring of the TELOS BPM are efficient and outcomes are evidenced-based. Evaluation contributes to the stability and sustainability of the model over time. Evaluation of physical, psychological, emotional, social, religious, spiritual, and cultural domains of end-of-life care provides the evidence for revision, refinement, and adjustment of the TELOS BPM to maximize patient and family outcomes. Evaluation of these components of well-being or human flourishing of persons is essential in order to develop and implement a plan of care that is authentic and patient-centered. The following practices are specific to the model's foundation in evaluation.

EVALUATION PRACTICES

Evaluation 1

Conduct both qualitative and quantitative research to provide evidence for the stability and sustainability of the BPM.

Evaluation 2

Construct an evaluation plan that tests the BPM over selected time frames.

Evaluation 3

Revise and update the model based on evaluative outcomes.

3.1 Consider eliminating a best practice that has proven ineffective, or just has no value to the patients and their families.

Evaluation 4

Evaluate knowledge of the TELOS BPM (available in Instructor Manual).

Evaluation 5

Evaluate confidence in performing best practices (available in Instructor Manual).

ECONOMICS PRACTICES

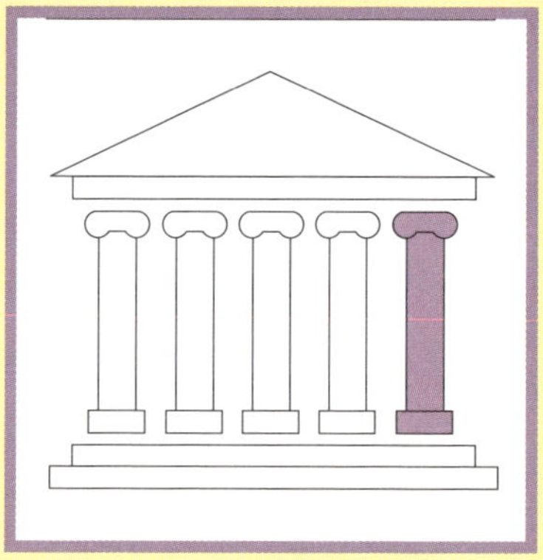

Economic support and administrative dedication to the TELOS BPM contribute to the stability and the sustainability of the model over time. Administrative support in an organizational climate that values the mission of, access to, and provision of quality care at the end of life is tantamount to the model's success in reducing the pain and suffering associated with trauma. Economic support in all the domains of end-of-life care including physical symptom relief as well as the health professionals' attention to the psychological, emotional, spiritual, religious, and cultural domains of care cannot be fragmented; no one domain has priority over the other, therefore, the economic support requires a holistic approach to patient care in order for it to be effective. The following practices are specific to the model's foundation in economics.

ECONOMICS PRACTICES

Economics 1

Ensure the funding of the TELOS BPM as part of the Trauma Program, e.g., through appropriate budgeting, partnerships with other community agencies, grants, and philanthropy.

Economics 2

Establish a budget that reflects the value of quality end-of-life care.

Economics 3

Give high priority to end-of-life care in terms of budgetary justifications.

3.1 Specified parking spaces for families who have been summoned to the emergency department in the event of a traumatic event or death of a loved one are justified based on the need for the family to have easy access to the emergency department in a timely fashion (in case the loved one is close to death).

3.2 Aesthetically pleasing designated rooms near the emergency department and the intensive care unit for family members of traumatically injured patients are justified by their needs for privacy, consultation with the healthcare team, and access to a restricted area for expressions of grief and pain.

3.3 ***Adequate staffing in the emergency department and intensive care unit is justified since it reflects the need for certain inter-professional team members to spend time with family members, to communicate with them on a timely basis, and to provide the needed psychological support as part of a holistic approach to care.***

Economics 4

Validate the value of quality end-of-life care.

4.1 Design and conduct research studies that measure the outcomes of the use of TELOS best practices.

4.2 Measure family satisfaction with end-of-life care.

4.3 Meet on a regular basis with interprofessional teams to monitor and evaluate their beliefs of how TELOS best practices have affected the quality of end-of-life care.

Economics 5

Engage administrators and management in the shared vision of the BPM.

INTRODUCTION TO PREHOSPITAL SETTING BEST PRACTICES

Best practices in this section are specifically for use in the prehospital setting. Practices from all environments may be integrated into various practice settings as indicated by the specific patient and/or family responses to the injury event. Please remember that the practices associated with the five pillars (engagement, ethics, education, evaluation, and economic practices) are to be considered when providing end-of-life care in any environment.

The Institute of Medicine (IOM) claims emergency medical services is at a *"crossroads,"* that hospital-based emergency care is *"at the breaking point"* and emergency care for children has *"growing pains."*[33] Over 40 years ago, trauma was cited as the *"neglected disease of modern society"* by the National Research Council.[34] Considerable federal funds were used to implement EMS systems across the country as a result of the federal EMS Act of 1973. Even though changes took place and strengths remain, a current IOM report[33] cites erosions of EMS systems. Cited problems associated with this *"national epidemic"* are overcrowded emergency departments and trauma centers, the change in the role of emergency departments for access to nonurgent health care, the congestion of intensive care units, and the problems with fragmented EMS systems. Of particular importance to the TELOS BPM is the problem of ambulance diversion as a reflection of the overcrowding issue. The Centers for Disease Control has reported that 45% of emergency departments in the United States have at some time been on diversion status.[35] These impressive trends support the concern of the appropriateness of transporting patients with no likelihood of survival to trauma centers and implementing aggressive resuscitation efforts either in the field or in the emergency department.

Guidelines[36-37] for withholding or withdrawing resuscitation from certain trauma victims have enormous implications for EMS personnel. They need to understand the reasons these guidelines were formulated and to understand the implications they may have for those on scene other than the victim. Transportation of the traumatized dead to a morgue or a new type of facility may be the right action to take. However, acceptance of the public will be necessary for such a change to take place. In our survey, 41% of the public in our survey preferred the morgue vis-à-vis the hospital where dead-on-scene victims be taken and 29.4% would accept such a new facility if religious and counseling services were available.[11] These are substantial percentages and may indicate that the change from transporting either dead traumatized patients or those for whom resuscitation has been withheld or withdrawn in the field to other facilities may be an option acceptable to the public.

Rarely do EMS personnel respond to a traumatic event and find no other persons at the scene but the victim. The primary responsibility of EMS personnel is to evaluate, provide care, stabilize, and most often transport the victim(s) to a trauma center. When the American Trauma Society refers to the 1st Trauma, they are referring to care of patients; when they refer to the 2nd Trauma, they are recognizing that there are typically other persons at the scene of a traumatic event and often these persons are members of the victim's family.[13] Recognizing that trauma affects the victim and his/her family, the following best practices are aimed at being attuned to the needs of both victims and families on scene. All victims are inextricably part of an environment of relationships and engagement with others; such engagement has implications for thoughtful, caring, and compassionate respect from EMS personnel. The practices are divided into sections related to; 1) general practices, 2) withholding/withdrawing practices, and 3) notification of death practices.

PREHOSPITAL GENERAL PRACTICES

Prehospital 1

Provide emergency trauma care according to your level of prehospital training and certification to all victims of trauma regardless of age, pre-existing diseases, or social distinctions.

Prehospital 2

Identify the patient, determine his/her identity, and if other family members are present, determine their identity and relationship to the patient.

Prehospital 3

Introduce yourself and what you are planning to do in order to foster trust.

Prehospital 4

Determine whether family members can cope with staying with a severely traumatized or expired trauma patient during your assessment and treatment.

4.1 Utilize other on-scene personnel, e.g., police, fire, other first responders, other family members, to escort a distraught family member away from the treatment area.

Prehospital 5

Consider transporting a close family member with the patient in the ground ambulance or helicopter, according to established protocols of your EMS service.

Prehospital 6

Provide the name of the destination hospital and directions to family members.

6.1 Instruct them to follow all traffic laws and speed limits.

6.2 Inform them not to follow you since you may pass through intersections and red stop lights (using safe driving skills).

WITHHOLDING AND/OR WITHDRAWING RESUSCITATION PRACTICES

All victims of trauma, regardless of age, pre-existing diseases, or social distinctions should have access to competent health professionals. These professionals should be skilled in emergency medical care in the prehospital setting and provide care with the intent of saving lives and transporting victims to emergency departments designated as trauma centers. Cardiopulmonary resuscitation is one treatment that may not be indicated for certain trauma victims. Some victims, who demonstrate certain injuries or responses to those injuries, may, on occasion, not be resuscitated in the event that they are in cardiopulmonary arrest or in the event that the trauma was fatal at the time of the event.

Recommendations for EMS providers to follow in these circumstances are taken from *Guidelines for Withholding or Termination of Resuscitation in Prehospital Trauma Cardiopulmonary Arrest* developed by the National Association of EMS Physicians (NAEMSP) Standards and Clinical Practice Committee and the American College of Surgeons Committee on Trauma.[36-37] The following specific recommendations for withholding or terminating resuscitation <u>do not</u> pertain to: 1) pediatric patients (less than 18 years of age), 2) patients in whom a medical cause such as a myocardial infarction is the likely inciting event, and 3) patients with complicating factors, such as the potential for severe hypothermia. Some states have adopted their own state guidelines related to prehospital resuscitation of trauma victims, for example, the Connecticut EMS Medical Advisory Committee (CTEMSMAC) has promulgated similar guidelines to national guidelines through the Office of Emergency Medical Services of the Connecticut Department of Public Health.[38] In circumstances of traumatic cardiac arrest associated with *"lightning strikes, drowning or hypothermia,"* Connecticut's guidelines recommend that resuscitation be initiated and the patient be transported to a hospital.[38]

Note

The following practices, *Prehospital 7-20,* are from the *Guidelines for Withholding or Termination of Resuscitation in Prehospital Traumatic Cardiopulmonary Arrest*[36-37] developed by the NAEMSP Standards and Clinical Practice Committee and the American College of Surgeons Committee on Trauma. Additional guidelines or reference to guidelines in the State of Connecticut *(see Appendix 3)* are so noted.[38]

Prehospital 7

Use all resuscitative measures including CPR for **clinically dead** trauma patients unless contraindicated by the exceptions listed below in *Prehospital 8*.

Prehospital 8

Withhold resuscitation from those trauma patients who are found to have no respirations and no carotid pulse in the following situations[36-37]:

8.1 Patient has a valid do-not-resuscitate (DNR) bracelet or DNR Transfer Form that:

8.1.1 conforms to the state specifications, color, and construction

8.1.2 is intact; it has not been cut or broken

8.1.3 is on the wrist or ankle

8.1.4 displays the patient's name and his/her physician's name

This practice *(Prehospital 8.1)* is specific to the State of Connecticut[38] *(see Appendix 4)*.

8.2 Patient shows signs of **decomposition**, **putrefaction**, decapitation, **hemicorporectomy**,[36-37] or **incineration**[38] (incineration is specific to the State of Connecticut).

8.3 *National guidelines recommend "resuscitation efforts should be withheld in victims of penetrating or blunt trauma with evidence of a significant time lapse since pulselessness, including dependent **lividity**, **rigor mortis**, and decomposition."*[37]

8.4 However, in the State of Connecticut, if the patient is assessed to have lividity, rigor mortis, or injuries incompatible with life (such as "*massive crush injury, complete exsanguination, severe displacement of brain matter*"), the following additional assessment is required <u>before</u> withholding resuscitation:[38]

8.4.1 "*Reposition the airway and look, listen, and feel for at least 30 seconds for spontaneous respirations; respiration is absent.*"

8.4.2 "*Palpate the carotid pulse for at least 30 seconds; pulse is absent.*"

8.4.3 "*Examine the pupils of both eyes with a light; both pupils are non-reactive.*"

8.4.4 Document lack of cardiac activity, in at least two leads, for at least 30 seconds[38] (if the EMS personnel are Advanced Life Support [ALS] providers) or

8.4.5 Document absence of a shockable rhythm for 30 seconds if an automatic external defibrillator (AED) is being used by Basic Life Support (BLS) providers.

8.4.6 Resuscitate those patients with lividity and/or rigor mortis if they are victims of hypothermia, lightning strike, or drowning.[38]

8.5 Patient has been pronounced dead at the scene in person by a licensed Connecticut physician or registered nurse.

8.6 Patient at a mass casualty incident is declared clinically dead prior to arrival in the treatment area.

Prehospital 9

"Resuscitation efforts may be withheld in any blunt trauma patient who, based on out-of-hospital personnel's thorough primary patient assessment, is found apneic, pulseless, and without organized electrocardiographic (ECG) activity upon arrival of emergency medical services (EMS) at the scene."[37]

9.1 Requires Medical Control approval in Connecticut.

Prehospital 10

***"Victims of penetrating trauma found apneic and pulseless by EMS, based on their patient assessment, should be rapidly assessed for the presence of other signs of life, such as pupillary reflexes, spontaneous movement, or organized ECG activity."*[37]**

10.1 Initiate resuscitation and transport the victim to the nearest emergency department or trauma center if any of these signs are present.

10.2 "*If these signs of life are absent, resuscitation efforts may be withheld*"[37] (requires Medical Control approval in the State of Connecticut).

Prehospital 11

Initiate CPR to the cardiopulmonary arrested patient "*in whom the mechanism of injury does not correlate with the clinical condition, suggesting a non-traumatic cause of arrest.*"[37]

Prehospital 12

***"Termination of resuscitation efforts should be considered in trauma patients with EMS witnessed cardiopulmonary arrest and 15 minutes of unsuccessful resuscitation and cardiopulmonary resuscitation."*[37]**

Prehospital 13

Individualize the guidelines and protocols for traumatic cardiopulmonary arrested patients who are transported.

13.1 Give consideration to factors such as the average transport time within the EMS system, the scope of practice of the various EMS providers, and the definitive care capability, i.e., trauma centers within the system to determine the receiving hospital.

13.2 Provide airway management and intravenous line placement when possible during transport to avoid extended on-scene time.

Prehospital 14

Be familiar with the guidelines and protocols affecting the decision to withhold or terminate resuscitation efforts.

14.1 "*Consider the needs of survivors when considering the discontinuation of a resuscitation, especially if crisis management may be needed.*"[38]

14.2 "*Scene management and safety of the crew and public may prevent withholding/discontinuation of resuscitation. In general, do not cease resuscitation in public places/establishments.*"[38]

14.3 Document "*all encounters with the patient's family, personal physician, scene physician or nurse, medical examiner, law enforcement,*" and Medical Control.[38]

Prehospital 15

Develop and implement all resuscitation withholding or termination protocols under the guidance of the EMS system's medical director.

Prehospital 16

Include information regarding notification of the appropriate law enforcement agencies and notification of the medical examiner or coroner for final disposition of the body in policies and protocols for termination of resuscitation efforts.

Prehospital 17

Provide EMS personnel with access to resources for debriefing and counseling as needed.

Prehospital 18

Monitor the adherence to policies and protocols governing the withholding or termination of resuscitation through a quality review system.

Prehospital 19

Provide the family members of persons who have died in the prehospital environment specific contact information for community resources to support them in their bereavement, including support that may be offered by local hospice units or hospitals.

Prehospital 20

Obtain medical control advice, as indicated by protocols, when implementing *Guidelines for Withholding or Termination of Resuscitation in Prehospital Traumatic Cardiopulmonary Arrest.*[36-37]

Prehospital 21

Explain futility, as indicated, and that resuscitative efforts are not indicated for those persons whose injuries were fatal on scene or for whom (according to the above guidelines) resuscitation is being withheld or withdrawn to those family members or significant others who are on scene with the patient.

Prehospital 22

Respect the pre-existing state regulations or law related to DNR orders of persons who reside in the community, e.g., skilled nursing facility, group home, who sustain a traumatic event while in that community dwelling *(see Appendix 4).*

22.1 Contact medical control using EMS protocols to inform him/her that the patient has a pre-existing DNR order.

Prehospital 23

Respect pre-existing state regulations or laws pertaining to clients of state agencies, e.g., Department of Developmental Services or Department of Mental Retardation *(see Appendix 5).*

NOTIFICATION OF DEATH PRACTICES

Prehospital 24

Develop a specific plan to notify families of the death of a family member on scene.

Prehospital 25

Provide families on scene with important information, e.g., telephone number of medical examiner's office (if that is the disposition of the body), receiving hospital's address/telephone number, and directions to the hospital (if that is the disposition of the body of a deceased victim).

Prehospital 26

Provide family members of persons who have died in the prehospital environment with:

26.1 any specific information about the disposition of the body

26.2 the address and phone number of the agency that will be receiving the body and the time frame in which such disposition will most likely occur

INTRODUCTION TO EMERGENCY DEPARTMENT BEST PRACTICES

Best practices in this section are specifically for use in the emergency department. Practices from all environments may be integrated into various practice settings as indicated by the specific patient and/or family responses to the injury event. Please remember that the general practices (engagement, ethics, education, evaluation, and economic practices) are to be considered when providing end-of-life care in any environment.

Visits to emergency departments increased 26% from 1993 to 2003 during a time when there was a net loss of 425 hospital emergency departments.[33] This impressive trend supports the concern of the appropriateness of transporting patients with no likelihood of survival to trauma centers and implementing aggressive resuscitation efforts either in the field or in the emergency department. This trend also poses concern for the availability of time of the health professionals and staff in emergency departments to spend with patients who have died (or expected to die in the emergency department) and their families. Conversations with families of victims who have died in the emergency department require time, attention, and compassion and such time is at a premium in overcrowded hospital settings that pull the health professionals away from these sensitive and painful situations. In one study "obstacles" to providing end-of-life care in the emergency department were identified as: 1) *"too high a workload to allow for adequate time to care for dying patients and their families,"* 2) *"having to deal with angry family members",* 3) *"poor design of emergency departments that do not allow for privacy of dying patients or grieving family members,"* 4) *"family members not understanding what 'life-saving measures' really mean,"* 5) *"not enough time to provide quality end-of-life care because the nurse is consumed with activities that are trying to save the patient's life."*[39] All of these *"obstacles"* are addressed in the following best practices in the emergency department.

Regarding care that the injured victim might receive in the emergency department, most respondents in our public and professional surveys would prefer to be in the treatment area while their loved one is being resuscitated. This is even more likely if the injured is a child. These preferences of the public and the professionals have implications for trauma professionals, especially trauma surgeons, many of whom would prefer that family members not be present. Reasons for not wanting families in the resuscitation room should be explored and policies and procedures decided in advance to reconcile these different preferences. Guidelines from the *National Consensus Conference on Family Presence During Pediatric Cardiopulmonary Resuscitation and Procedures* have been agreed upon by a number of major professional organizations, including the American College of Surgeons to offer and support **family presence** during resuscitation of children.[40] Emergency department best practices are divided into sections related to: 1) communication practices, 2) family presence practices, 3) decision-making practices, and 4) **death and dying** practices.

COMMUNICATION PRACTICES

Emergency Department 1

Contact family members (not present at the time of admission of a loved one) by telephone to inform them that the patient is in the emergency department.

1.1 Educate those professional staff authorized to make such calls in communication skills specifically for this practice.

1.1.1 Rehearse and practice making this kind of phone call.

1.1.2 Use a clear and calm voice, speak slowly and distinctly, use an introductory sentence that prepares the recipient of the call, e.g., "*Your daughter (name) was involved in a serious accident.*"[13]

1.1.3 Be aware of the Health Insurance Portability and Accountability Act (HIPAA, 1996) as related to discussing Personal Health Information (PHI).[24]

1.1.4 Be familiar with the policies and privacy practices of your institution related to patients' rights regarding privacy of their PHI.

1.1.5 Be familiar with any exceptions to disclosure of PHI of a trauma victim related to special laws or rules for psychiatric, drug and alcohol, or HIV-related protected information.

1.2 ***Know the name of the patient, extent of the injuries, the circumstances of the traumatic event, and the current condition of the patient before calling the family.***

1.3 Conduct the conversation in a quiet private area to reduce any interruptions.

1.4 Do not convey news of a traumatic event or traumatic death on a voicemail or answering machine. Leave a message for the person to call you back.

1.5 ***Do not inform family members of a death over the telephone. Wait until they arrive in the emergency department so an appropriate relationship can be established and support services have been assembled.***

1.5.1 Acknowledge a death truthfully only if the family member asks if the patient has died.

1.5.2 Determine if the contact person is the most appropriate family member, e.g., spouse or parent of victim.

1.5.3 Determine if the contact person is alone in case the call incapacitates him/her, so that emergency medical services or police can be notified.

1.5.4 Determine if the call is being received on a cellular phone while the contact is driving; if so, suggest that he/she drive to a safe area off the road and stop the car for the conversation.

1.5.5 There may be exceptions to informing relatives over the telephone of the death of a loved one, e.g., relatives who live out of state or are traveling away from home.

1.5.5.1 Attempt to determine their distance away and if necessary, inform them of the death in a compassionate manner.

1.5.5.2 Communicate a preamble sentence that prepares the relative for bad news, e.g., *"I have some disturbing news about your son."*

1.5.5.3 Ask the relative if he/she is alone and suggest he/she contact someone to stay with him/her.

1.6 Communicate clearly and succinctly which hospital is calling, directions to the hospital if needed, where to park when they arrive, where to go once they arrive, who will meet them, and that the physician will speak with them upon their arrival.

1.6.1 It is recommended that a specific parking area be designated for families being called to the emergency department in the event a loved one has been injured.

1.7 Reinforce that the trauma team is with the patient and that all care is being provided.

1.8 Provide the direct emergency department phone number to the person who is being notified.

1.9 Identify and document on a family notification form:

- *1.9.1* name of the person who contacted the family
- *1.9.2* name and relationship to the patient of the person to whom information was given over the telephone
- *1.9.3* time of the call
- *1.9.4* whether or not anyone from the family is coming to the hospital

Emergency Department 2
Identify family members once they arrive at the hospital and establish a particular person as the family contact person.

Emergency Department 3
Avoid asking for insurance information early on in the relationship with the family of a patient who has been critically traumatized.

Emergency Department 4
Provide continuous information to the family regarding the patient's condition.

4.1 Communicate with the family, when possible, by having the physician leader in charge of the patient's care talk to the family, e.g., the senior trauma surgeon.

4.2 Communicate with the family at regular intervals throughout the patient's resuscitation and stay in the emergency department, using the same person, if possible.

4.3 Designate this person as the **support person** between the family and the healthcare team.

- *4.3.1* Provide the family initially with basic information such as the patient's location, the name of the attending physician caring for the patient, and a general explanation of injuries sustained, and let them know that more precise information will be forthcoming from the physician.
- *4.3.2* Gather any information about the patient from the family that may contribute to the care the patient is receiving, e.g., pre-existing medical conditions, current medications the patient may be taking.

4.4 ***Be aware that "minutes seem like hours" to family members who are waiting anxiously for information.***

Emergency Department 5

Disclose to family members the prognosis and the likelihood of the patient's survival.

Emergency Department 6

Inform the family if death is likely utilizing the following practices:

6.1 Communicate with the family if you are the physician team leader.

6.2 Explain, according to the detail known, the circumstances of the injury event.

6.3 Explain the injuries and reason for impending death.

6.4 Involve the family in goal-of-care decisions.

6.5 Communicate medical, physiologic futility if present, prognosis of death, and continuity of comfort care.

6.6 Encourage all team members to support the information given to the family by the physician team leader to foster consistency in information.

Emergency Department 7

Inform the family of a patient's death in a compassionate and caring manner.

7.1 ***The senior physician in charge of the patient's care should inform the family of the patient's death.***

7.2 Designate a space in the emergency department where families can gather to have conversations with healthcare team members as related to the death of a patient.

7.3 Use the following guidelines of the American Trauma Society to tell a family that a loved one has died in the emergency department[13]:

7.3.1 collect all information pertinent to the patient's death; know the cause of death

7.3.2 change into a lab coat that is clean and blood-free

7.3.3 determine the patient's first name

7.3.4 know where the body is and where and when the family can view the body

7.3.5 request that you not be disturbed during the conversation with the family

7.3.6 be accompanied by another health professional who can support the family

7.3.7 introduce yourself, your role in the patient's care, and identify the relationship to the patient of those family and friends present

7.3.8 follow *Engagement Practices 5-10*

FAMILY PRESENCE PRACTICES

Emergency Department 8

Consider family presence during resuscitation and during the administration of life-saving care as an option for family members on a case-by-case basis.[40,41]

8.1 Give special consideration when the victim is a child since many parents want to be present when their child is seriously injured and/or when death is likely.[11]

8.2 Offer family presence as an option when the care to the patient will not be interrupted and after an assessment of family members wishing to be present. Assess for[40]:

- *8.2.1* combative and threatening behavior
- *8.2.2* extreme emotional volatility
- *8.2.3* behaviors consistent with intoxication or altered mental status
- *8.2.4* disagreement among family members
- *8.2.5* threat to the safety of the healthcare team

8.3 ***Designate a staff professional as the support person for the family member who wishes to be in the resuscitation room to monitor the family member's response and to guide behavior.***

8.4 Prepare and instruct the family member(s) who wants to be present in the resuscitation room with an explanation of the following:

- *8.4.1* actual appearance of the patient and what to expect in the resuscitation room
- *8.4.2* description of procedures being performed

8.5 Establish the following agreements with those close family members who request presence in the resuscitation room to facilitate the process. Family members must agree to:

8.5.1 follow the instructions of the identified support person who will remain with them during their presence in the resuscitation room

8.5.2 stand in a place decided by the support person so that no interruptions in the medical and nursing care will occur

8.5.3 leave the room when requested by the support person as indicated by the family member's response or the team's request

8.5.4 follow the support person's guidance as to how to provide comfort to the patient

8.6 Recognize that some physicians and other health professionals may not agree with family being present in the resuscitation room.

8.6.1 Construct a plan as to how to address these concerns in advance.

DECISION-MAKING PRACTICES

Emergency Department 9
Provide emergency care to all patients who are not responsive based on the principle of **presumed consent**.

Emergency Department 10
Determine the patient's capacity to make healthcare decisions.

Emergency Department 11
Determine the appropriate surrogate if the patient does not have the capacity to make his/her own healthcare decisions.

11.1 Determine the capacity for the surrogate to be a valid surrogate, one who is free of conflicts of interest and who provides convincing evidence of knowledge of the patient's values and preferences.

Emergency Department 12
Determine if the patient has advance directives, e.g., living will, designation of a healthcare representative.

Emergency Department 13

Utilize a shared decision-making model to include the family in the treatment decisions that respect the values and beliefs of the patient and are in the patient's best interest.

Emergency Department 14

Determine options for care based on an assessment of biological objective data, e.g., diagnostic laboratory determinations, physiological measurements, and effectiveness of treatment in conjunction with subjective values and overall expectations of benefit (determined by patient and/or family/surrogates) and burdens such options may incur.

14.1 Refer to *Ethics Best Practice 21 and 22* related to medical futility.

Emergency Department 15

Respect the patient's **advance directive** as, and if, it pertains to the current injury event.

15.1 According to Connecticut law, a living will may address *"any kind of health care you may receive. Should one be in a **terminal condition** or **permanently unconscious**, the living will can also tell your physician when you want life support systems to keep you alive or whether you do not want to receive such treatment."*[42] Either of these may be difficult to determine in the emergency department setting. Although the Patient Self-Determination Act is a federal mandate, individual states are responsible for implementing the act and pertinent legislation may differ from state to state.

15.2 If the living will is "*hopelessly ambiguous*"[43] and you cannot determine its applicability to the current patient situation, explain to the patient's surrogate decision maker that you appreciate his/her providing the living will but for now you and he/she should proceed to shared decision making.

15.3 Determine the patient's prior health status and use this information to make decisions about the patient's goals of care following the traumatic event.

15.4 Identify the reason why a family member is requesting to not invoke an existing advance directive (if applicable), and determine its validity.

15.5 ***Acknowledge your moral and legal obligation to respect an advance directive that is appropriate to follow in this particular situation.***

15.6 Use conflict resolution or ethics consultation if decisions of family members are inconsistent with the best medical judgment of the physicians caring for the patient.

Emergency Department 16
Determine the patient's organ donation status.

DEATH AND DYING PRACTICES

Emergency Department 17
Consider discontinuing resuscitation efforts being performed on victims who meet the criteria outlined in the practices described in *Prehospital 7-20*.

Emergency Department 18
Recruit nurses, social workers, or patient advocates to provide emotional and psychological support of the family when the patient is critically ill or has died.

Emergency Department 19
Assess the patient's and family's spiritual needs and provide interventions to meet those needs.

19.1 Respect the family member's belief in Divine Intervention if such a belief is determined.

Emergency Department 20
Identify specific values, beliefs, and rituals of different cultures that require the healthcare team's sensitivity and attention during the dying process and after death.

Emergency Department 21
Provide a private and respectable room for an expired patient so that the family may view the body and engage in initial bereavement.

Emergency Department 22
Provide physical care to the patient that optimizes the patient's appearance to the family, e.g., grooming the patient while being cognizant of the need to follow hospital policies related to what can and cannot be done to the body postmortem, positioning him/her in a position of perceived comfort, covering injuries to reduce stress to the family.

Emergency Department 23
Have a list of funeral homes and their phone numbers by town readily available for families.

Emergency Department 24
Assist family members, once they have viewed the body of their loved one (if desired), to leave the hospital; answer any questions, explain the forthcoming process for disposition of the body, provide psychological support, and provide them with a contact phone number if they have additional questions.

Emergency Department 25
Provide family members with the hospital's resources or other resources for bereavement.

INTRODUCTION TO INTENSIVE CARE UNIT BEST PRACTICES

Best practices in this section are specifically for use in the intensive care unit. Practices from all environments may be integrated into various practice settings as indicated by the specific patient and/or family responses to the injury event. Please remember that general practices (engagement, ethics, education, evaluation, and economic practices) are to be considered when providing end-of-life care in any environment.

Once a trauma patient is in the intensive care unit and there is a possibility that the patient may die from his/her injuries, there are particular issues faced by intensive care unit health professionals that are somewhat different from dealing with possible death of a nontraumatized patient. The suddenness and acuity of the trauma event, the critical nature of the injuries, the overwhelming feelings of guilt that families of victims often experience, the need to make immediate life and death medical decisions, and the unfamiliarity with the values and preferences of persons at the end of their lives due to trauma result in end-of-life scenarios that pose unique situations requiring unique practices.

Every effort is made to heal an injured patient and typically trauma patients require time in the intensive care unit for the magnitude and consequences of their injuries to be manifested. However, if it is determined that choices regarding goals of care need to be made, this decision process should be one that is shared by the interprofessional team and those persons who are considered valid surrogate decision makers for the patient in the event the patient does not have capacity to make his/her own health decisions. Results of our surveys of health professionals and the general public demonstrated that, if injured, most preferred that they be made comfortable rather than have everything possible done to keep them alive in the event that death is likely.[11] However, when the same question was asked regarding decision making for a loved one, the percentages dropped.[11] This may indicate that persons have a harder time selecting an option for a focus on comfort for their loved ones than for themselves.

In cases where doctors believe that there is no hope of recovery, most respondents in our survey supported the withdrawal of **life-sustaining treatments** and a change in focus to comfort care.[11] However, of those who prefer continuing all efforts indefinitely, the majority of the public believes that these efforts should continue regardless of the financial cost. When efforts will take medical resources and personnel away from individuals who are more likely to survive, the majority of respondents believe life-sustaining efforts for those with no hope of recovery should not continue.[11] This may indicate that the public and professionals support the need to achieve fair and just use of scarce resources.

When respondents were asked specifically about circumstances of medical futility, the majority indicated that the patient should be made as comfortable as possible, aggressive treatment should be stopped, palliative care continued, and life support removed.[11] Most indicated that they trust a doctor's decision to stop life-saving treatment when such treatments are determined to be overall medically futile. However, most of the public respondents believed that Divine Intervention could save someone despite what the physicians may think.[11] While physicians can be reasonably sure that they are trusted to make decisions regarding futility, they need to be prepared to deal with families who are waiting for a miracle. Similarly, most of the public respondents believe that a person in a persistent vegetative state (PVS) can be saved by a miracle. However, if they were ever in a PVS, greater than 80% of the public and professional respondents would prefer to die.[11]

A large percentage of the public respondents believed that they have the right to demand care that doctors think will not help.[11] Because of this entitlement belief, conflicts regarding providing care that physicians have judged is physiologically futile often arise when patient's families demand care in the hopes that "everything be done" for their loved one to save his/her life. Practices to resolve these conflicts related to futility are included in the following section.

Half of the public and almost 80% of the professionals reported that they are potential organ donors.[11] Over 85% of the respondents in both groups believe that their family should not be able to reverse their decision to donate their organs.[11] This has profound implications for organ donation and the professionals who deal with families of donors. If a patient meets the legal and medical criteria as an organ donor, his/her wishes should be honored. Families who disagree with the patient's preference will need support and counseling if organ procurement occurs without their approval. Letting families know that most people do not want their decision to be reversed may lessen their angst about organ donation.

The public and the professional respondents in our study felt the same about living wills; family members should not be able to change their living will.[11] This information may help families respect and abide by the preferences and wishes previously stated by trauma victims prior to their injury events. The results of our survey are reflected in the following best practices for care in the intensive care unit: 1) admission and discharge practices, 2) communication practices, 3) decision-making practices, 4) physical symptom management practices, and 6) death, dying, and withdrawal of life-support practices.

ADMISSION AND DISCHARGE PRACTICES

Intensive Care Unit 1

Establish a plan for implementation of intensive care unit admission and discharge criteria that do not depend on bed availability, but depend upon the appropriateness of intensive care to meet the needs of the patient and coincide with the agreed upon level of care required *(see Intensive Care Unit 13)*.

1.1 Admit patients to the intensive care unit based on pre-established criteria.

1.2 Transfer patients out of the intensive care unit who no longer meet the criteria for staying in the intensive care unit in order to keep beds available for incoming trauma victims who need intensive care and meet the criteria for admission.

1.3 ***No patient should stay in the intensive care unit who does not meet admission criteria simply because the bed is available.***

1.4 Transfer a patient to a designated palliative care bed or palliative unit when the focus of care for the patient has been determined, through shared decision making with the family and healthcare team, to be focused on comprehensive palliation.

Intensive Care Unit 2

Orient the patient, if possible, and the family members to the intensive care unit environment, e.g., visiting practices, telephone number and any practice, such as a voice mail system, of when and who to call, important logistical information, such as lodging, if needed.

Intensive Care Unit 3

Have available the following printed materials for family members available from the Society of Critical Care Medicine[44]:

3.1 Common Problems of Critical Illness

3.2 What Are My Choices Regarding Life Support?

3.3 Participating in Care: What Questions Should I Ask?

3.4 Taking Care of Your Self While a Loved One is in the ICU

3.5 Making Decisions About ICU Care

3.6 Why Do ICU Patients Look and Act That Way?

COMMUNICATION PRACTICES

Intensive Care Unit 4

Utilize an interprofessional team model to formulate, clarify, revise, and then consistently communicate the goals of care.

4.1 Meet as an interprofessional team to discuss goals of care that have been decided, the patient's physical condition, as well as the patient's responses in other domains, i.e., psychological, social, spiritual, cultural.

4.2 Construct a plan of communication with family members that fosters a team approach and avoids clinical services giving different messages about the patient to the family; coordinate how conversations with family members are conducted. Individual clinical services should communicate to other interprofessional team members their conversations with families so that communications are shared and prognoses that are given are similar.

4.2.1 Such conversations should be recorded in writing on a special intensive care unit form *(see Appendix 6)* designed for such purpose *(Intensive Care Unit 8)*.

Intensive Care Unit 5

Provide the patient and family consistent, accurate, and reliable information.

5.1 Initially provide information that describes the mechanism of injury (e.g., motor vehicle crash, fall, gunshot), extent of the injuries sustained, description of anticipated medical interventions, treatments, and any operative plans.

5.2 Describe reasonable expectations of the patient's course; avoid unrealistic expectations while maintaining hope if the prognosis is uncertain.

5.3 Avoid giving a precise prognosis of <u>when</u> the patient will die, if death is expected, unless it is quite predictable; use appropriate ranges if it will be minutes, hours, or days. Communicate that any prediction is only an estimate and cannot be determined with certainty.

5.4 Identify the medical specialty teams that are involved in the patient's care, e.g., orthopedics, neurosurgery.

5.5 Identify the intensive care unit staffing pattern, e.g., role of the intensivist physician in the patient's care, primary nursing if available, role of advanced practice nurses and/or physician assistants.

Intensive Care Unit 6

Provide continuity of care by assigning the same healthcare team members since typically the length of stay of a trauma patient in the intensive care unit is short.

6.1 Adjust staffing and medical rotations to facilitate such continuity.[45]

Intensive Care Unit 7

Consider <u>not</u> using "team rounds" as a time to have family members be involved in learning about and participating in the patient's plan of care.

7.1 Discuss the benefits and burdens of including family members on routine *"rounds"* with the healthcare team before implementing such a practice.

7.2 <u>Benefits</u> may include:

- *7.2.1* having the family members participate in deciding options of care that are based on their values and beliefs
- *7.2.2* the family perceives they are an active part of their loved one's treatment
- *7.2.3* easy access to the healthcare team
- *7.2.4* access to detailed reports of the patient's trajectory postinjury

7.3 <u>Burdens</u> may include:

- *7.3.1* Focusing on the patient as an *"object"* of care rather than a *"subject"* in his/her own life narrative where diagnostic and laboratory data become central to defining the patient's condition.
- *7.3.2* Families are conforming to the *"system"* and power remains with the system.
- *7.3.3* Families may become overwhelmed with technical jargon and not comprehend the meaning of certain terms; rounds are not in a *"language"* that family members are accustomed to hearing and they may be reluctant to participate in the role of family member.
- *7.3.4* The intent of rounds is interprofessional collaboration and education; families should not have to participate in this forum to garner information and share their wishes (use other communication strategies to achieve these objectives that place the family's concerns first).

7.3.5 There may be conflicts between healthcare team members that need to be addressed without the family being present.

7.3.6 Rounds have a teaching agenda in trauma centers and this educational forum may not be appropriate for family member involvement.

7.4 Have nurses and social workers available to address any burdens that may occur as a result of family members attending rounds.

7.5 Establish reasonable behavioral expectations of family members and healthcare team members if and when family members are a part of rounds.

7.5.1 Explain to family members during their orientation to the intensive care unit, that families are invited to attend rounds with healthcare team members and that questions and clarification of any issue are encouraged.

7.5.2 Explain the goal of such rounds, the role of members of the team who may attend, and the expected time frame for conducting rounds.

7.5.3 Discuss with family members the process of rounds and their role in this process.

Intensive Care Unit 8
Provide access to critical patient information to all healthcare team members.

8.1 Utilize a standardized form that is immediately recognizable to healthcare team members that includes:

8.1.1 specific goals of care as determined and agreed upon by the patient or surrogate and attending physician in conjunction with the health care team *(see Levels of Care in Intensive Care Unit 13)*

8.1.2 patient's advance directives and resuscitation status

8.1.3 name and contact information of the designated surrogate

8.1.4 all diagnoses, prognoses, and updates told to which family member and on what date

8.1.5 identification of specific healthcare team members who provided the information *(Intensive Care Unit 8.1.4)*

8.1.6 write bulleted information and avoid lengthy narrative notes, but maintain accuracy and thoroughness of information provided

Intensive Care Unit 9

Communicate to the family and/or surrogates that death has occurred when a patient has been declared brain dead.

9.1 Communicate the fact of **brain death** to the family or surrogate in a compassionate and succinct way.

9.1.1 Certain family members may not accept the concept of brain death, especially when the patient has cardiac activity; explain in simple terms that brain function has ceased and that such cessation is legally an indication of death.

9.2 ***Removal of any life-sustaining treatment from a patient who has been declared brain dead is the responsibility of the health care team and does not necessitate consent from family members or valid surrogates.***

DECISION-MAKING PRACTICES

Intensive Care Unit 10

Continue the trauma surgeon's involvement as the main contact with the patient and family to maximize shared decision making and the fiduciary relationship.

Intensive Care Unit 11

Determine the goals of care, and develop and document a comprehensive plan of care that includes pain and symptom management, resuscitation status of the patient, and the valid surrogate for the patient who lacks capacity to make healthcare decisions.

11.1 Determine the goals of care through a shared decision-making model that sees both the family and healthcare team as having input into decisions regarding treatment.

11.2 Support the goals of care when they have been decided based on a consensus of the majority; do not sabotage their implementation if you do not agree with them and do not communicate your opposing view to the patient's family.

11.3 Engage the gold standard of advanced care planning (early discussion and planning for possible events, e.g., need for artificial ventilation, medical hydration and nutrition) early in the patient's admission so that values and preferences of the patient and/or family can be heard initially in the admission.

Intensive Care Unit 12

Initiate discussion with surrogates in the event that it is the physician's best medical judgment that the patient has a low likelihood for survival and further curative, aggressive treatment is physiologically futile.

12.1 If the family disagrees with a physician's medical judgment, other interprofessional team members should be apprised of the reasons for the controversy in order to be fully informed for conversations with the interprofessional team and the family.

12.2 However, do not challenge, in a disdainful manner, a family's wish to continue care by saying, *"Why are you doing this?"* when you as a member of the healthcare team feel aggressive care is inappropriate and may be causing harm to the patient.

12.2.1 Start a conversation by saying, *"The physician has told you that this situation is very grave and that he/she recommends palliative care only; let's talk about what you are thinking right now."*

Intensive Care Unit 13

Offer and describe appropriate and medically indicated **levels of care** based on the patient's condition.

13.1 Level One care is continuation of all aggressive care and implementation of new aggressive care, including CPR, for treatment of any new onset problems.[46]

13.2 Level Two care is continuation of selective aggressive care with or without resuscitation, if needed, but with continued life-sustaining and palliative care.[46]

13.3 Level Three care is continuation of life-sustaining care, palliative care, and current aggressive care but no escalation of care for any new problems and typically no cardiopulmonary resuscitation.[46]

13.4 Level Four care is continuation of palliative care with withdrawal or withholding of life-sustaining care and injury-specific, curative, or aggressive care.[46]

Intensive Care Unit 14

Consider using the VALUE mnemonic during meetings with families; V represents valuing and appreciating what the family members are saying, A represents acknowledging the emotions of family members, L represents listening to family members, U represents understanding the patient as a person, and E represents eliciting questions from family members.[47]

Note: When the VALUE method was tested in a randomized controlled study in twenty-two ICUs with families of 126 patients, families exposed to family meetings that were longer and used the principles of the VALUE mnemonic scored significantly lower in measures of stress, depression, and impact of event scales 90 days after the family meeting.

14.1 Ensure that all health professionals who attend a family meeting are current as to the patient's condition and the goals of the meeting prior to the meeting.

14.2 Utilize the resources of designated health-informed interpreters since family members who are acting as interpreters for other family members may misinterpret medical information.[48]

14.3 End a family meeting or conference reviewing the decisions that were made.

14.4 Diffuse the burden of decision making as it may overwhelm a particular family member.

Intensive Care Unit 15

Determine options for care based on an assessment of biological objective data, e.g., diagnostic laboratory determinations, physiological measurements, and effectiveness of treatment in conjunction with subjective values and overall expectations of benefits (determined by patient and or family/surrogates) and burdens such options may incur.

Intensive Care Unit 16

Offer only those interventions or treatments that achieve the established goal of care.

16.1 ***Do not offer CPR to those patients for whom scientific and empirical evidence has proven that it is not medically indicated, will offer no effect, and is not indicated based on medical standards of care and is therefore considered physiologically futile.***

16.1.1 Offering CPR to a patient for whom the physician has determined that CPR is not medically indicated, will offer no benefit, and is not based on medical standards of care may cause unnecessary burden to the patient's family.

16.1.2 Determine if your state has a legal requirement for consent from a surrogate for a DNR order for those patients for whom CPR is not medically indicated.

16.1.2.1 In the event that conflict arises in this situation, request an ethics consult.

16.2 Do-not-resuscitate orders for clients of the Connecticut Department of Mental Retardation (DMR), now referred to as the Department of Developmental Services (DDS) in Connecticut, have specific guidelines that must be followed *(see Appendix 5)*.

Intensive Care Unit 17

Recognize that families and surrogates need a reasonably sufficient time to decide what is in the patient's best interest.

17.1 Avoid pressuring surrogates (family next-of-kin) to make decisions.[3]

17.1.1 Decide beforehand the person to discuss code status with families to avoid having the family or surrogate feel badgered by multiple persons approaching them.

17.2 Avoid using phrases that minimize the shared decision-making process, such as *"What do you want us to do?"* or *"You tell us when you want us to stop."*

17.3 Acknowledge the problem that certain patients may not be appropriate for prolonged intensive care unit stays, the so-called *"lingering in the intensive care unit"* phenomenon[46]

17.3.1 Reinforce the reality of the likelihood of death or poor outcome, as needed.

17.3.2 Avoid conveying unrealistic expectations of survival.

17.3.3 Recognize that asking families to make difficult decisions at the end of life for their suffering family member is often an unbearable burden.

17.3.4 Lessen the above burden with compassion, lamentation, and straightforward recommendations.

Intensive Care Unit 18

***Recognize that there is no moral obligation to provide care that in one's best medical judgment is medically futile.*[49]**

18.1 In the event that family members or surrogates demand care that the physician deems medically futile or contraindicated, the physician should discuss his/her judgments with those who are making decisions for the patient.

18.2 In the event the family members or surrogates continue to demand such care, obtain a second medical opinion.

18.3 In the event that the second medical opinion concurs with the first opinion, and the family members or surrogate still demand such care, obtain an ethics consultation.

18.4 In the event that the ethics consultation leads to an agreement with the family that the care demanded is not futile, attempt to transfer the patient to another physician who is willing to assume the responsibility of the patient's care.

18.5 In the event that the ethics consultation leads to an agreement with the physicians that the care demanded is futile, the family should be notified that the patient will be transferred to another facility within a reasonable time to obtain such a transfer agreement.

18.6 Refer to the hospital's futility policy for the process of resolving conflicts related to futile care conflicts.

Intensive Care Unit 19

Keep all conversations regarding futility focused on securing the patient's good.[30]

Intensive Care Unit 20

Identify the caregiver who is most trusted by the patient and family; invite this person to be present at all conversations about treatment options.[30]

Intensive Care Unit 21

Assess the patient from three perspectives[30]:

21.1 current health state of patient

21.2 influence of this state on the patient

21.3 influence on the patient's ability to achieve meaningful life goals

Intensive Care Unit 22

Be sensitive to professional and societal factors that contribute to futility conflicts.

Intensive Care Unit 23

Help the family or surrogate to separate the patient's suffering from their suffering.

23.1 Be careful to notice when family or surrogates are focusing more on how they are suffering.

23.2 Shift the conversation to the patient's best interests and concerns.

23.3 Do not minimize suffering of the family or surrogate; yet keep focused on making decisions that are in the best interests of the patient instead of how medical decisions will affect family or surrogate decision makers.

Intensive Care Unit 24

Respect and honor a patient's organ donation preference.

24.1 If the patient is registered as an organ donor in the State of Connecticut Organ Donor Registry, this autonomous choice of the patient is morally and legally obligatory to follow.

24.2 ***A family's or surrogate's consent is preferred but not required to proceed with organ donation from a trauma victim who is registered with the Organ Donor Registry in Connecticut and whose circumstances meet the criteria for organ donation.***

24.2.1 Psychological attention to the needs of those family members or surrogates who do not agree with the patient's autonomous choice to be an organ donor is essential to reduce suffering and anguish.

24.3 Facilitate early access to organ procurement services, if that is the decision made.

PHYSICAL SYMPTOM MANAGEMENT PRACTICES

Intensive Care Unit 25

Use standards of care for physical symptom management, e.g., pain, restlessness, dyspnea, agitation.

25.1 Assess and plan interventions that relieve physical symptoms.

25.2 Communicate the above plan with all members of the interprofessional team.

25.3 Document those interventions that are implemented, their effects, and their modification, if indicated.

25.4 Use standards of care for pharmacological, nonpharmacological, and alternative methods that have proven effectiveness.[50-52]

25.5 Other physical symptoms experienced by patients at the end of life who are dying from a terminal disease, e.g., cancer, are rarely issues for the trauma patient at the end of life. However, if they do occur, terminal restlessness, anorexia, cachexia, ascites, bladder spasms, bowel incontinence, bowel obstruction, constipation, diarrhea, and dyspnea are physical symptoms that require thoughtful, empirically proven interventions depending on the etiology of the symptom and the proximity to death.[53]

Intensive Care Unit 26

Assure the family that any physical suffering the patient may experience will be immediately assessed and appropriate interventions will be taken to promote physical comfort.

Intensive Care Unit 27

Request a palliative care consult if needed.

DEATH, DYING, AND WITHDRAWAL PRACTICES

Intensive Care Unit 28

Orchestrate a plan for withdrawal of life-sustaining treatments that meets the needs of families to participate in the process in a way that recognizes their values and preferences.

28.1 ***Designate a nurse, once the decision has been made to withdraw life-sustaining care, as the primary team member to orchestrate, plan, and implement those plans for withdrawal of life-sustaining care.[54]***

Note: Nursing philosophy of caring, engagement, and healing is the foundation for nurses assuming the responsibility of orchestrating withdrawal plans with the family and other interprofessional team members.

28.1.1 The patient's physician should have an active role in the withdrawal plans.

28.2 Do not give any impression that the patient is being abandoned.

28.3 Recognize and be sensitive to the role of the interprofessional team members as *"moral strangers"*[55] to the families at this extraordinarily personal and private time of the death of their family member.

28.4 Provide physical care to the patient that optimizes the patient's appearance to the family during those *"final hours or moments"* of life by keeping the head of the bed slightly elevated to avoid patient drooling, by grooming the patient, and by positioning him/her in a position of perceived comfort.

28.5 Minimize family's anxiety during the withdrawal process by reducing external stimuli, e.g., reduce harsh lighting, minimize the sounds of technology, and provide undisturbed privacy.

28.5.1 Support any family member who does not want to be present for withdrawal of life support. Do not try to persuade or coerce any family member who decides that being present for the withdrawal is too painful to experience.

28.6 Explain to the family what will happen during the withdrawal process.

28.6.1 Assure the family that any symptoms of discomfort, anxiety, or distress of any kind will be managed by the healthcare team.

28.6.2 Do not give precise predictions regarding the time between withdrawal of life support and death; these times are unpredictable.

28.6.3 Determine through caring communication whether family members are interested in a very detailed explanation of the withdrawal process or whether a more general less detailed explanation better meets their needs.

28.6.4 Determine whether family members prefer to be alone with their loved one or whether they would find more comfort from having professional team members present; such determination comes with experience and a sense of the moment.

28.6.5 Collaborate with a senior health professional if you are involved in withdrawal of life support for the first time or if you feel that you need advice from an experienced mentor.

28.7 Identify and support the family's preferences for rituals related to dying, e.g., clergy present, ability to surround the patient's bed, chanting, ceremonies, displaying of religious symbols.

28.7.1 Assess and determine the safety of any requested ritual.

28.7.2 Prohibit the use of any ritual that has a risk of injury.

28.7.3 In the event safety is jeopardized, explain and justify why the ritual is prohibited and offer and explore an alternative.

Intensive Care Unit 29

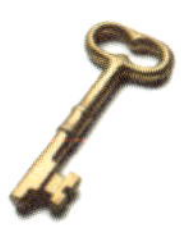

Avoid the premise that health professionals are "allowing" families to implement their preferences during the dying process or that families have to ask "permission" to implement a preference. As long as there is no threat to safety, such preferences should simply be facilitated.

Intensive Care Unit 30

Avoid delaying the withdrawal of life-sustaining treatments for extended periods of time after the decision has been reconciled by the healthcare team and the family members who are present.

30.1 Waiting for the arrival of other family members prior to withdrawal for an extended period of time (e.g., longer than 8-12 hours) may put undue stress on those family members who are present and may put a disproportionate burden on the resources of the intensive care unit.

30.2 The practice of waiting extended periods of time is not in the best interest of the patient but may assuage the suffering and discomfort of family members not present who want to be; decide on a case-by-case basis.

30.2.1 Any delay must be morally justifiable.

30.2.2 Obtain an ethics consult if family is requesting a delay greater than 12 hours.

30.3 Remove life-sustaining support, e.g., artificial ventilation, from those patients who have been declared brain dead.

30.3.1 Consent to remove life-sustaining support from a patient who has been declared brain dead is not required from the family or surrogate.

30.3.2 Remove life support after proper and timely notification of the family, giving them reasonable time to be present, if they so desire.

30.3.3 Do not delay removal of life support from brain dead patients for extended periods of time to wait for other family members to arrive; this is disrespectful to the expired person.

30.3.4 There is no reasonable moral justification for utilizing intensive care unit physical resources and personnel to provide prolonged postmortem care to brain dead patients.

REFERENCES AND NOTES

1. Heron, M., Hoyert, D. L., Murphy, S. L., Xu, J., Kochanek, K. D., Tejada-Vera, B. (2009). Deaths: final data for 2006. National Vital Statistics Reports 57(14). US Department of Health and Human Services, Centers for Disease Control and Prevention, National Center for Health Statistics, National Vital Statistics System. Available at: http://www.cdc.gov/nchs/data/nvsr/nvsr57/nvsr57_14.pdf. *Accessed March 19, 2009.*

2. Clarke, E. B., Curtis, J. R., Luce, J. M., et al. (2003). Quality indicators for end-of-life care in the intensive care unit. *Critical Care Medicine, 31* (9), 2255-2262.

3. Siegel, M. D. (2009). End-of-life decision making in the ICU. *Clinics in Chest Medicine, 30,* 181-194.

4. Aristotle (trans. 1962). *Nicomachean ethics* (Translated by Ostwald). Englewood Cliffs, NJ: Prentice Hall.

5. Pellegrino, E. D. (2001). Philosophy of medicine: Should it be teleologically or socially constructed? *Kennedy Institute of Ethics Journal, 11*(2), 169-180.

6. Carse, A. L. (2006). Vulnerability, agency, and human flourishing. In C. Taylor & R. Dell'Oro (Eds.), *Health and human flourishing* (pp.33-52). Washington, DC: Georgetown University Press.

7. Boal, A. (2000). *Theatre of the oppressed* 2nd ed. (Translated by C. A. and Leal McBride & E. Fryer). London: Pluto Press.

8. Boal, A. (2002). *Games for Actors and Non-actors* 2nd ed. (Translated by Adrian Jackson). London: Routledge.

9. Torke, A. M., Quest, T. E., Kinlaw, K., Eley, J. W., Branch, W. T. (2004). A workshop to teach medical students communication skills and clinical knowledge about end-of-life care. *Journal of General Internal Medicine, (19),* 540-544.

10. Barnett, K. G., & Fortin, A. H. (2006). Spirituality and medicine: A workshop for medical students and residents. *Journal of General Internal Medicine, (21),* 481-485.

11. Jacobs, L. M., Burns, K., Bennett Jacobs, B. (2008). Trauma death: Views of the public and trauma professionals on death and dying from injuries. *Archives of Surgery, 143*(8), 730-735. Copyright© 2008 American Medical Association. All rights reserved.

12. Gadow S. (1999). Relational narrative: The postmodern turn in nursing ethics. *Scholarly Inquiry for Nursing Practice: An International Journal, 13* (1), 57-69.

13. Cronin, M., Kelly, P., McQuay, J., Scott, J., Sise, M., Teter, H. (2006). *The 2nd trauma program: The art of communicating with families of trauma patients.* Maryland: American Trauma Society.

14. Olson, J. K., & Kunyk, D. (2004). Empathy. In S. J. Peterson & T. S. Bredow (Eds.), *Middle range theories* (pp. 151-164). Philadelphia: Lippincott Williams & Wilkins.

15. Prendergast, T. J., & Puntillo, K. A. (2002). Withdrawal of life support: Intensive caring at the end of life. *Journal of the American Medical Association, 288* (21), 2732-2740.

16. Purnell, L. D., & Paulanka, B. J. (2005). *Guide to culturally competent health care.* Philadelphia: F. A. Davis.

17. Marshall, P. L., & Koenig, B. A. (2001). Ethnographic methods. In J. Sugarman & D. Sulmasy (Eds), *Methods in medical ethics* (pp. 169-191). Washington, DC: Georgetown University Press.

18. Koenig, B. A., & Gates-Williams, J. (1995). Understanding cultural difference in caring for dying patients. In Caring for patients at the end-of-life [Special Issue]. *Western Journal of Medicine, 163*, 244-249.

19. Sulmasy, D. P. (2006). Spiritual issues in the care of dying patients. *Journal of the American Medical Association, 296* (11), 1385-1392.

20. Taylor, C. (2007). Values, ethics & advocacy. In C. Taylor, C. Lillis, P. LeMone (Eds), *Fundamentals of nursing* (6th ed.). Philadelphia: Lippincott, Williams, & Wilkins.

21. Pellegrino, E. (1979). The anatomy of clinical judgment. In H. T. Engelhardt, S. F. Spiker, B. Towers (Eds.). *Clinical judgment: A clinical appraisal* (pp. 169-194). Holland: Kluwer Academic Publishers.

22. Sulmasy, D. P. (2000). Healing the dying: Spiritual issues in the care of the dying patient. In D. C. Thomasma & J. L. Kissell (Eds.). *The health care professional as friend & healer* (pp. 188-197). Washington, DC: The Georgetown University Press.

23. Beauchamp, T. (1999). Failure of theories of moral personhood. *Kennedy Institute of Bioethics Journal, 9* (4), 309-324.

24. The following is from the American Trauma Society's book, *The 2nd Trauma Program: The Art of Communicating with Families of Trauma Patients.*

"The American Trauma Society (ATS) requested and received legal opinion in response to the question, 'When a patient with a serious injury is in an emergency care facility, may the trauma team notify the family of the patient's location and status and if so, to what extent?' Under HIPAA, a health care provider may disclose PHI [personal health information] *to a patient's friends and family including family members, other relatives, or close, personal friends of the patient. The health care provider may also disclose PHI to entities that will notify or assist in the notification of a patient's family and friends, such as the police. The amount of PHI that may be disclosed varies depending on the scope of consent given by the patient or the amount of relevant PHI required for particular disclosure purpose."* (See Reference 13, ATS, 2006, p. 9).

25. Pellegrino, E.P., & Thomasma, D.C. (1993). *The virtues in medical practice.* New York: Oxford University Press.

26. Webster, G. C., & Baylis. F. (2000). Moral residue. In S.B. Rubin & L. Zoloth (Eds), *Margin of error: The ethics of mistakes in the practice of medicine*. Hagerstown, MD: University Publishing Group.

27. Singer, P.A., Pellegrino E.P., & Siegler M. (2001). Clinical ethics revisited. *BMC Medical Ethics, 2* (1), 1-8.

28. Bennett Jacobs, B., & Taylor, C.R. (2006). Medical futility from the natural attitude. *Advances in Nursing Science, 28* (4), 288-305.

29. Pellegrino, E.D. (2000). Decisions to withdraw life-sustaining treatment: A moral algorithm. *Journal of the American Medical Association, 283* (8), 1065-1067.

30. Taylor, C. (1995) Medical futility and nursing. *Journal of Nursing Scholarship, 27* (4), 301-306.

31. Education in Palliative and End-of-Life Care (EPEC), Available at: http://www.epec.net

32. American Association of the Colleges of Nursing (AACN). *The End-of-Life Nursing Education Consortium* (ELNEC). Available at: http://www.aacn.nche.edu/elnec

33. Institute of Medicine of the National Academies. (2006). Committee on the Future of Emergency Care in the United States Health System Board on Health Care Services. *Hospital-based emergency care: At the breaking point.* Washington, DC: National Academies Press.

34. National Research Council of the National Academy of Sciences. (1966). *Accidental death and disability: The neglected disease of modern society.* Washington, DC: National Academy of Sciences.

35. Centers for Disease Control and Prevention. (2006). Quick stats: Percentage of hospital emergency departments (EDs) having to divert ambulances, by selected characteristics, United States, 2003. *Morbidity and Mortality Weekly Report, 55* (13), 372.

36. National Association of EMS Physicians (NAEMSP) Standards and Clinical Practice Committee and the American College of Surgeons Committee on Trauma. (2003). Guidelines for withholding or termination of resuscitation in prehospital traumatic cardiopulmonary arrest. *Journal of the American College of Surgeons, 196,* 475-481.

37. Hopson, L.R., Hirsh, E., Delgado, J., Domeier, R.M., McSwain, N.E. Krohmer, J. (2003). Guidelines for withholding or termination of resuscitation in prehospital traumatic cardiopulmonary arrest: A joint position paper from the National Association of EMS Physicians Standards and Clinical Practice Committee and the American College of Surgeons Committee on Trauma. *Prehospital Emergency Care, 7* (1), 141-146.

38. State of Connecticut, Department of Public Health (2009). *Guidelines for MRT, EMT - B, I, and paramedic. Determination of death/discontinuation of pre-hospital resuscitation for adults age 18 and over: Non-mass casualty situations.*

39. Heaston, S., Beckstrand, R., Bond, A., Palmer, S. (2006). Emergency nurses' perceptions of obstacles and supportive behaviors in end-of-life care. *Journal of Emergency Nursing, 32* (6), 477-485.

40. Henderson, D. P., & Knapp, J. F. (2006). Report of the national consensus conference on family presence during pediatric cardiopulmonary resuscitation and procedures. *Journal of Emergency Nursing, 32* (1), 23-29.

41. Mangurten, J., Scott, S.G., Guzzetta, C.E., Clark, A.P., Vinson, L., Sperry, J., Hicks, B., Voelmech, W. (2006). Effects of family presence during resuscitation and invasive procedures in a pediatric emergency department. *Journal of Emergency Nursing, 32* (3), 225-233.

42. Office of the Attorney General, State of Connecticut. (2006) *Your rights to make health care decisions: A summary of Connecticut law*. Available at: http://www.ct.gov/ag/lib/ag/health/yourrighttomakehealthcaredecisions2006version.pdf

43. Olick, R. S. (2001). *Taking advance directives seriously.* Washington, DC: Georgetown University Press.

44. Society of Critical Care Medicine. Available at: http://www.sccm.org

45. Clarke, E.B., Curtis, J. R., Levy, M., Danis, M., Nelson, J., Solomon, M. Z. (2003). Quality indicators for end-of-life care in the intensive care unit. *Critical Care Medicine,* 31(9), 2255-2262.

46. Huffman, J.L. (2002). Lingering in the intensive care unit. Palliative care by the surgeon. *Journal of the American College of Surgeons, 194* (4), 509-537.

47. Lautrette, A., Darmon, M., Megarbane, B., Joly, L., Chevret, S., Adrie, C., et al. (2007). A communication strategy and brochure for relatives of patients dying in the ICU. *New England Journal of Medicine, 356* (5), 469-478.

48. Crawley, L. M., Marshall, P. A., Lo, B., et al. (2002). Strategies for culturally effective end-of-life care. *Annals of Internal Medicine, 136,* 673-679.

49. Council on Ethical and Judicial Affairs (2008). *Code of medical ethics of the American Medical Association: Current opinions with annotations 2008-2009 edition.* Futile care opinion 2.035 and Medical futility in end-of-life care opinion 2.037. United States of America: American Medical Association.

50. Mackersie, R. C., Pittet, J. F., Dicker, R. A. (2008). Principles of critical care. In E. E. Moore, D. V. Felicano, K. L. Mattox (Eds), *Trauma,* (6th ed.) (pp. 1193-1224), New York: McGraw Hill.

51. Jacobi, J., Fraser, G. L., Coursin, D. B., et al. (2002). Clinical practice guidelines for the sustained use of sedatives and analgesics in the critically ill adult. *Critical Care Medicine, 30,* 119-141.

52. Quijada, E., & Billings, J.A. (2002). Fast facts and concepts #60 pharmacologic management of delirium: Update on newer agents. *End-of-life Physician Education Resource Center*. Available at: http://www.eperc.mcw.edu

53. Perry, P.H. (2005). *Core curriculum for the generalist hospice and palliative nurse*, (2nd ed.). Dubuque, Iowa: Kendall/Hunt Publishing.

54. Bennett Jacobs, B. (2002). *Surrounding death: A phenomenology of withdrawal of life support from trauma*. Unpublished Doctoral Dissertation. University of Connecticut, Storrs, Connecticut.

55. Engelhardt, H. T. (1996). *The foundations of bioethics*. New York: Oxford University Press.

56. Beauchamp, T. L., & Childress, J. F. (2009). *Principles of biomedical ethics*, (6th ed.). New York: Oxford University Press.

57. Quality Standards Subcommittee of the American Academy of Neurology (2010). Evidence-based guideline update: Determining brain death in adults. *Neurology, 74*, 1911-1918.

58. The Multi-Society Task Force on PVS. (1994). Medical aspects of the persistent vegetative state: first of two parts. *New England Journal of Medicine, 330* (21), 1499-1508.

59. The Multi-Society Task Force on PVS. (1994). Medical aspects of the persistent vegetative state: second of two parts. *New England Journal of Medicine, 330* (21), 1572-1579.

GLOSSARY OF TERMS

Abandonment – a breach of fidelity, trust, and any promises made to a patient; not attending to or continuing to treat a patient after establishing a relationship without informing patient. *(Ethics 14.1)*

Advance Directives – instructions left by persons when they had the capacity to make such instructions; in the State of Connecticut, advance directives take the form of a living will, or designation of a healthcare representative (Connecticut state-specific terms). Related to advance directives is The Patient Self Determination Act, a federal law effective in 1991 that mandates patients must be informed in writing upon admission of their right to accept or refuse treatment, their rights under existing state laws regarding advance directives, and the policies of the institution regarding the withholding or withdrawing of life-sustaining treatments. *(Emergency Department 15-16)*

Advanced Care Planning – the planning persons do prior to their actually becoming ill or injured. Such planning is the gold standard to establish one's values and preferences for treatments in the event such treatments would be required when they may not be capable of making their own healthcare decisions; it is recommended that such planning take place between persons, their family and primary care physician. *(Intensive Care Unit 11.3)*

Assent – typically refers to children who do not have the legal authority to make informed consent or refusal decisions but are said to be able to assent or dissent to procedures; although the child may not have the legal authority to make his/her medical decisions, it is recommended that the child's assent or dissent be determined based on their level of understanding of the procedure being suggested. *(Ethics 18)*

Autonomy – Greek *autos* is self and Greek *nomos* is rule—therefore autonomy refers to "*self-rule that is free from both controlling interference by others and from certain limitations such as inadequate understanding that prevents meaningful choice.*"[56] *(Ethics 2)*

Boalean Theater Forum – a sort of "*theatrical game*" that is a dramatization of a problem that is first presented by actors or role players and then members of an audience (spect-actors) can participate in the solving of the problem by substituting themselves on stage for the original actors.[7-8] *(The Best Practice Model)*

Brain Death – as defined by the American Academy of Neurology in 1995; three criteria to determine brain death are: coma or unresponsiveness, absence of brainstem reflexes, and apnea.[57] *(Intensive Care Unit 9.1)*

Caring Communication – communication between patients, families, and health professionals; such communication demonstrates to the receiver compassion, sensitivity, consistency, truthfulness, and is also timely. *(Engagement 8)*

Clinically Dead – *"any unresponsive patient found without respirations and without a palpable carotid pulse."*[38] *(Prehospital 7)*

Communicative Rapport – a useful and harmonious relationship; facilitates meaningful communication between patients, families, and health professionals. *(Engagement 7)*

Comportment (Ethical) – Ethical comportment or behavior is the result of the process of moral reasoning and is demonstrated by the actions and behaviors of moral agents using the elements of moral reasoning *(see Moral Agency)*. *(The Best Practice Model)*

Confidentiality – a patient's right that health care professionals will protect information and not disclose any information that they have disclosed to you *"in confidence."* *(Ethics 8)*

Consent or Refusal – the four elements of obtaining a consent or refusal from a patient for a particular treatment or intervention are: 1) duty to disclose the nature, purpose, risks, consequences, benefits, probability of success, feasible alternatives, prognosis with or without the intervention, 2) determination of decision-making capacity, 3) comprehension, and 4) voluntary decision making without persuasion or coercion. *(Ethics 16-18)*

Culture – acquired knowledge that people use to interpret experience and generate social behavior; the culture of a group is a social construction of concepts, beliefs, and principles of action and organization; as a group develops the knowledge to deal with external adaptation and internal integration, they build up patterns of basic assumptions that are handed down to newcomers to the group; culture is learned, not innate; socially acquired knowledge, traditions, lifestyles of a group; culture is a shared system that provides social structure for daily living, beliefs, values, habits, likes and dislikes, behavioral expectations, customs; culture is not an explanation for social behavior, people don't belong to cultures, people belong to groups, societies, or communities; it is often said that culture is what is *"between people."* *(Engagement 13-15)*

Death and Dying – death is an event; dying is a process. *(Engagement 25)*

Decision-Making Capacity – the patient's ability to understand information necessary to make any one decision at any one point in time, ability to reason in accord with a relatively consistent set of values, ability to communicate preferences; competence is a related legal term. *(Ethics 16.2)*

Decomposition or Putrefaction – *"the skin is bloated or ruptured, with or without soft tissue sloughed off. The presence of at least one of these signs indicated death occurred at least 24 hours previously."*[38] *(Prehospital 8.2)*

Dignity – the value and worth of persons; persons have such worth because of their moral standing as human beings who, when rational and with critical mental capacities, have the freedom from external constraints to determine their own aims. Intrinsic dignity or the dignity one has as a human being cannot be *"lost"* or eradicated; persons die with intrinsic dignity always. Attributed dignity is the dignity that others show or attribute to persons. By attributing dignity to a person, a health professional is respecting that person's intrinsic dignity. Attributing dignity to persons is often what is compromised when one is ill or injured. *(Ethics 3)*

Economics – a way of using science (social) to study a particular good or service, in this case the provision of end-of-life care to trauma victims and their families, by evaluating the production, distribution, source, demand, and price of the service. *(Economics Introduction)*

Education – teaching and learning activities to enhance the knowledge of health professionals involved in end-of-life care of trauma victims and their families; such activities include initial programs to describe the TELOS best practices, as well as continuing education activities to refine and keep knowledge of TELOS up-to-date.

ELNEC – *The End-of-Life Nursing Education Consortium.* Available at: www.aacn.nche.elnec. A project of the Association of the American Colleges of Nursing, which trains ELNEC educators to disseminate knowledge through a modular course in end-of-life care for nurses. *(Education 7)*

Empathy– understanding another's thoughts and feelings and communicating that understanding to them. *(Engagement 7.6)*

Engagement – the mutual indebtedness between patients and health professionals is the foundation for the patient/health professional relationship. *(Engagement Introduction)*

EPEC – *Education in Palliative End-of-Life Care.* Available at: www.epec.net. A project originally funded by the Robert Wood Johnson Foundation, with multiple learning modules available online or through conferences around the country. *(Education 6)*

Ethics – Clinical ethics is the identification, analysis, and solving of problems with moral relevance that arise in the clinical setting. *(Ethics Introduction)*

Ethics of Care – a theory of ethical reasoning that has as its core the importance of relationships, their contextual importance, and the patient's personal narrative; issues of trust, bonding, love, and inter-relational contingency are important in reflecting on moral dilemmas using the ethics of care approaches. *(Engagement Introduction)*

Ethnicity – a group's heritage, including language, dialect, religious practices, literature, music, folklore, political interests, food preferences, and employment patterns. *(Engagement 2)*

Evaluation – the process needed to ensure that the development, implementation, testing, and monitoring of the TELOS BPM are efficient and outcomes represent evidenced-based care and values-based practice. *(Evaluation Introduction)*

Existential Concerns or Existential Suffering – each person is constituted by his existence to *"be"* or to exist; each person determines his/her aims and goals; value and meaning of life, hopes, fears, purpose, afterlife beliefs, guilt, and forgiveness are frequent existential concerns of dying persons; as opposed to physical suffering, i.e., pain. Patients who are existentially suffering are concerned for and asking questions about meaning and value of life; families may also existentially suffer when a loved one is injured and dying. *(Engagement Introduction)*

Family Presence – family members who are physically present in the actual resuscitation room or treatment room during the treatment or resuscitation of a loved one. *(Emergency Department 8)*

Fidelity – staying true to one's word; acting in good faith to keep promises to patients; abandonment is a breach of fidelity. *(Ethics 13)*

Fiduciary Relationship – the relationship between patients and health professionals based on trust. *(Engagement 2)*

Futility – medical futility is determined by evaluating the effectiveness, benefits, and burdens of a particular treatment. A physician can determine that a particular treatment has no <u>effect</u>, or in other words, will not achieve its physiologic goal or alter the patient's overall anticipated course. Patients (or surrogate decision makers) determine <u>benefits</u> of treatments by evaluating the treatment's value and desirability as they perceive such value subjectively. <u>Burdens</u> of treatments are determined by both physicians and patients (or surrogate decision makers); burdens related to facts are determined by a physician, burdens related to subjective and personal issues of the patient are determined by the patient (or surrogate decision makers).[29] Quantitative futility (often referred to as the fact distinction in futility discussions) refers to the inability of a particular treatment that is not medically indicated to offer effectiveness for the patient. Qualitative futility (often referred to as the value distinction in futility discussions) refers to the inability of a particular treatment to offer benefit to the patient. *(Ethics 21-22; Intensive Care Unit 18-22)*

Hemicorporectomy – *"transection of the torso; the body is completely cut across below the shoulders and above the hips through all major organs and vessels. The spinal column may or may not be severed."*[38] *(Prehospital 8.2)*

Human Flourishing – a concept related to *"well-being"* whereby a person experiences the *goods* of life and experiences well-being in the following domains: interpersonal, material, physical, self-determination, social inclusion, and rights. *(Engagement Introduction)*

Incineration – *"90% of body surface area 3° burn as exhibited by ash rather than clothing and complete absence of body hair with charred skin."*[38] *(Prehospital 8.2)*

Interprofessional Team – professionals, e.g., nurses, doctors, social workers, pastoral care representatives, who share common concerns to achieve the goals of care of a patient using a shared conceptual framework that respects their individual disciplines while at the same time recognizes the need for coordination of care through a team approach. *(Engagement 4; Ethics 10)*

Intersubjective Contingency – the relationship between a patient and a health professional is one of respect for the existential nature of those persons involved or respect for the uniqueness of each person in the relationship. *(Engagement Introduction)*

Justice – what the individual health professional owes to each patient is commutative justice or giving a patient his/her due, in other words, persons have rights to fair and equal treatment; the question of what goals should guide resource allocation and how goals should be achieved through fair and equitable distribution are the issues involved with distributive justice. *(Ethics 23-24)*

Latino or Hispanic – according to the US Census Bureau, those people who classify themselves in one of the following categories: Mexican, Mexican American, Chicano, Puerto Rican, or Cuban, as well as those who indicate that they are *"other Spanish/Hispanic/Latino,"* including those whose origins are from Spain, the Spanish-speaking countries of Central or South America, the Dominican Republic, or people identifying themselves generally as Spanish, Spanish American, Hispanic, Hispano, or Latino. Origin can be viewed as the heritage, nationality group, lineage, or country of birth of the person or the person's parents or ancestors before their arrival in the United States. *(Appendix I ICU Scenario Two)*

Levels of Care – Level One care is continuation of all aggressive care including implementation of new aggressive care, including CPR, for treatment of any new-onset problems. Level Two care is continuation of selective aggressive care with or without resuscitation, if needed, but with continued life-sustaining and palliative care. Level Three care is continuation of life-sustaining care, palliative care and current aggressive care but no escalation of care for any new problems and typically no resuscitation. Level Four care is continuation of palliative care with withdrawal or withholding of life-sustaining care and injury-specific, curative, or aggressive care.[46] *(Intensive Care Unit 13)*

Life-sustaining Treatments – those medical interventions or treatments that support a person's physiological functions only, e.g., mechanical ventilation for respiration, artificial hydration and nutrition for water and nutrient needs; in contrast to therapeutic or curative treatments that are intended to treat or cure a particular malady. *(Engagement 11.1.2)*

Lividity with rigor mortis – *"when clothing is removed, there is a clear demarcation of pooled blood within the body, and the body is generally rigid."* This does not apply to victims of lightning strikes, drowning, or hypothermia.[38] *(Prehospital 8.3)*

Moral Agency – one's elements of being an agent of action; moral agency elements include: 1) character or habitual predispositions (virtues) that contribute to how one acts as a moral agent, 2) valuing or determining those values that contribute to moral actions, 3) sensibility or being able to recognize a moral moment matters, 4) responsiveness or responding to the challenges that the moral moment presents, 5) reasoning or determining the justifications and distinctions to explain the action one takes, 6) discernment or using character and values to morally reason through the moment to come up with an action that is based on moral theory, principles, codes, etc., 7) accountability or taking responsibility for moral actions and one's recommendations to others, 8) advocacy and leadership or going beyond the single moral moment to think about whether the particular moral action is broader and more comprehensive than the current situation at hand, e.g., making changes within an organization so that the environment is conducive to ethical moral behavior and comportment.[20]

Moral Distress – when one's held beliefs or values are inconsistent with one's actions; often can result when social, organizational, or institutional constraints do not support or acknowledge what one believes is the right thing to do, resulting in doing something that is not in accordance with one's own moral code.[26] *(Ethics 14.1.5)*

Moral Residue – *"that which each of us carries with us from those times in our lives when in the face of moral distress we have seriously compromised ourselves or allowed ourselves to be compromised."*[26] *(Ethics 14.1.5)*

Palliative Care – supportive, comfort care in the context of trauma refers to the comprehensive care provided to a patient for whom aggressive, curative, or technical interventions are not indicated; comprehensive palliative care includes attention to the physical, psychological, and spiritual needs of the individual patient. *(Engagement 11.1.3)*

Permanently Unconscious – According to changes in Section 19a-570 of the Connecticut General Statutes (CGS) related to living wills, permanently unconscious is defined as *"permanent coma and persistent vegetative state and means an irreversible condition in which the individual is at no time aware of himself or the environment and shows no behavioral response to the environment."*[42] *(Emergency Department 15.1)*

Persistent Vegetative State (PVS) – a clinical condition, according to the American Academy of Neurology; persons in a PVS are unaware of self and their environment; accompanied by sleep-wake cycles with either complete or partial preservation of hypothalamic and brainstem autonomic functions; no evidence of ability to interact with others; no evidence of sustained, reproducible, purposeful, or voluntary behavioral responses to visual, auditory, tactile, or noxious stimuli; no evidence of language comprehension or expression; bowel and bladder incontinence; variable preserved cranial and spinal reflexes.[58-59] *(Intensive Care Unit Introduction)*

Presumed Consent – the justification for providing necessary and emergency care to those patients who do not have decisional capacity or are unresponsive and need procedures that are necessary and the risk would be too great to wait for the patient to gain decisional capacity, to regain consciousness, or to locate an appropriate surrogate decision maker. *(Emergency Department 9)*

Privacy – ethically speaking, privacy is a right of patients that protects their liberty to be in a private *"zone"* that by its nature is protected from intrusion by others. Health professionals ought to protect patient's privacy by delineating a zone inhibiting the intrusion of persons not associated with the patient's care or persons the patient has not consented to be involved. *(Ethics 7)*

Prudential Question in Clinical Ethics – What is the <u>right</u> (based on scientific standards and empirical evidence) and <u>good</u> (based on the patient's values and preferences) action to take that is in the best interest of the patient? *(Ethics 1)*

Putrefaction or Decomposition – *"the skin is bloated or ruptured, with or without soft tissue sloughed off, or there is the odor of decaying flesh. The presence of at least one of these signs indicated death occurred at least 24 hours previously."*[38] *(Prehospital 8.2)*

Race – according to the US Census Bureau, the five races include American Indian or American Native, Asian, Native Hawaiian or Pacific Islander, Black or African American, and White. *(Engagement 2)*

Shared Decision Making – making decisions about patients' goals of care and treatments that respect the patients' values, preferences, and autonomy without compromising the integrity of health professionals; involves sharing such decision making with patients, families, surrogate decision makers, and health professionals. *(Ethics 9; Intensive Care Unit 11.1)*

Spiritual Concerns of the Dying – such concerns are questions patients and their surrogate decision makers may have related to value, as in human dignity, and meaning of life, as in hope (in this case, "*ultimate hope*" or a "*transcendental object*"); Sulmasy explains that "*the opposite of hope is despair but despair is really just another name for meaninglessness; to suffer without any sense of meaning is abject hopelessness; health care professionals do not give their patients dignity or hope. Dignity and hope are already present as givens in every situation of death. Value is already there, commanding respect. Meaning is already there, awaiting affirmation. The task of the health care professional is to show respect and reverence for the dignity that all dying persons have simply because they are human, and to share their own hope that meaning transcends the dying process.*" [22] *(Engagement 16-24)*

Support Person – the person in the emergency department who is designated to stay with the family of a critically injured or expired patient to act as a liaison between the family and healthcare team to provide updated, accurate, and consistent information regarding the patient's condition. This person may also be the designated individual to stay with those family members who wish to be present in the resuscitation room. *(Emergency Department 8.3)*

Surrogate – someone who can validly represent another's values and preferences and who is designated or appointed to make decisions for a patient who does not have the capacity to make his/her own decisions; surrogates ought to possess healthcare decision-making capacity, be free of conflicts of interest, and give convincing evidence of knowledge of the patient's values and preferences (if a person unrelated to the patient is appointed by a court, such person may not know the patient and therefore may not know the patient's values and beliefs). *(Engagement 1)*

TELOS – acronym for *Trauma End-of-Life Optimum Support*. TELOS is a Greek word for end or purpose of something; in this sense, the purpose of the practice of health professionals engaged with trauma victims is caring, comfort, and ultimate healing. Teleology, in a philosophical sense, is in contrast to philosophical naturalism, meaning that teleology or the belief that things in nature have a purpose first, such as humans have a purpose to hear and therefore have ears (form follows function), is contrasted to naturalism or the belief that function follows form, for example, that hearing is because humans have ears. Healing, comfort, and caring are the purposes (form) of the patient/health professional relationship (function). *(The Best Practice Model)*

Terminal Condition – According to the Connecticut General Statute related to advance directives, a terminal condition *"means the final stage of an incurable or irreversible medical condition which, without the administration of a life support system, will result in death within a relatively short time, in the opinion of the attending physician."* (This definition in Section 19a-570 of the Connecticut General Statutes (CGS) was effective as of October 1, 2006). *(Emergency Department 15.1)*.[42]

Types of Care – three types of care include: 1) injury-specific, disease-specific, aggressive curative care, 2) life-sustaining care that supports life's physiological functions only, e.g., mechanical ventilation, artificial hydration and nutrition, 3) palliative, supportive, comfort care in the context of trauma refers to the comprehensive care provided to a patient for whom aggressive, curative, or technical interventions are not indicated; comprehensive palliative care includes attention to the physical, psychological, and spiritual needs of the individual patient. *(Engagement 11.1)*

Veracity – telling the truth; obligation to tell the truth is based on respect for others. *(Engagement 8.1)*

Virtues of Health Professionals – moral character that reflects the habitual predispositions of fidelity to trust and promise, benevolence, effacement of self-interest, compassion, caring, intellectual honesty, justice, prudence, or practical wisdom; whether or not these virtues can be taught is an interesting philosophical question. *(Ethics 13)*

Withholding/withdrawing – withdrawing is discontinuing a treatment already started, e.g., mechanical ventilator; withholding is not initiating a particular treatment. *(Prehospital 7-21; Intensive Care Unit 28-30)*

APPENDIX 1

SCENARIOS FOR ROLE PLAY OR BOALEAN THEATER FORUM

INTRODUCTION

These scripted scenarios may be used for conventional role-play and are also conducive to Boalean Theater Forum. Boalean Theater Forum is an adaptation of theater developed by Augusto Boal who founded the Theater of the Oppressed. The actors (health professionals acting *qua* health professional or *qua* patient or family) perform a play with a script. At any point during the play, any "spect-actor" from the audience attending the educational program may clap his/her hands and call out "stop!" then take the place of the actor portraying any one individual already on the "stage." In other words, those in the audience listening to the script are not just idle spectators (audience) but can participate in the action on stage as "spect-actors." As Boal stated:

> Communication between actor and audience takes place at two levels: 'wave' and 'underwave' or 'undercurrent.' Actors communicate to an audience on a conscious level, by means of the thoughts they 'emit.' When an actor's thoughts are not in accord with his action – i.e., when there is a clash between wave and undercurrent – the audience/receiver experiences a phenomenon similar to interference on the radio; the audience receives two contradictory messages and it is impossible to register them both.[8]

The objective of this technique is to respect the "other's" view of how to approach a particular situation using, in this case, TELOS Best Practices. An additional objective is to recognize and respect the voices of the many "players" involved in difficult situations that arise at the end-of-life.

The following are hypothetical situations encountered in the prehospital setting, emergency department, or intensive care unit setting. The scenarios describe the individuals who interact in each situation.

Throughout each scenario, there are italicized comments that relate what is being said to the best practices presented in TELOS. Reading through the scenarios and comments provides one way to deal with the situations using TELOS best practices. These scenarios can be used as a basis for role play to rehearse the principles taught in a TELOS course or as a starting point for a Boalean Theater Forum.

Prehospital Scenario: Explaining to a family member or bystanders that an expired trauma victim does not meet the criteria for resuscitation.

Emergency Department Scenario One: Contacting a family member from the emergency department via telephone to tell him/her that a family member has just been brought to the emergency department in critical condition following a stabbing.

Emergency Department Scenario Two: Having a discussion between a nurse and a physician regarding family presence in the treatment/resuscitation room.

Intensive Care Unit Scenario One: Talking to a family about focusing the goals of care on comfort and less on aggressive/curative/injury-specific care.

Intensive Care Unit Scenario Two: Discussing medical futility with a patient's family.

SCENARIO FOR ROLE PLAY OR BOALEAN THEATER FORUM FOR PREHOSPTIAL PROFESSIONALS

Explaining to a family member or bystanders on scene that an expired trauma victim does not meet the criteria for resuscitation

You arrive on the scene of a self-hanging of a young man in his early 20s. The neighbor spotted him from the yard and called 911. The curtains are partly open in the room, affording a view from the neighbor's yard. The victim lives with his mother who will be returning from work shortly. On attempting to call her, the police discovered she has left work for home.

The man was urgently cut down and was placed supine on his bedroom floor prior to your arrival. His arms are already stiff. Although it is difficult to move his head due to stiffening, you attempt to reposition the airway and from your assessment you determine that he is not breathing, has no pulse, and shows absolutely no signs of life; you determine that it is unknown how long he has been in this condition. An examination of his pupils shows no reflexes, no response to light, and they are fixed and dilated. There is venous congestion above the level of the bruising around his neck and there is evidence of blunt airway injury.

Determine if CPR should be initiated and if the patient needs to be transported to the hospital. Assess the patient using primary survey techniques to ascertain whether or not the patient is breathing and/or has a pulse; contact medical control.

At this moment there is a commotion at the door and a woman barges in, screaming.

Mother of the Victim
"Danny! Danny! What's going on here? Tell me he's OK!"

You turn and stand to meet her at the doorway to the bedroom.

Mother of the Victim
"I'm Daniel's mother," she frantically tells you. She sees her son over your shoulder and screams, "Danny!" then asks, "Why does his face look like that? You're going to take him to the hospital aren't you? He's going to be OK isn't he?"

You manage to get her out of the doorway, partially closing the door before finding her a chair.

Paramedic
"Mrs. Robertson, I am one of the paramedics who was called by your neighbor. I'm afraid I have some bad news. Your neighbor called us earlier. When we got here, we determined that your son was not breathing and his heart apparently stopped some time ago. There is nothing we can do to revive your son; Daniel is dead."

Allow silence for his mother to process what you have just told her.

Establish a communicative rapport when having conversations with family members. Introduce yourself and your role. Position yourself close to the family member, sit if possible and look the relative directly in his/her eyes when speaking; making a judgment as to whether touching would be perceived as appropriate. *(Engagement 7, 7.2, 7.5)*

Mother of the Victim
"What? No! That can't be!" Crying, "How do you know? Take him to the hospital now! It's the best in the state and they perform miracles there! They can save him!"

Paramedic
"Ma'am he was already dead when we found him. Our physical exam has confirmed that." ***Allow silence again.*** "There is nothing we can do to try and bring him back." ***Maintain eye contact.***

Listen to the response of the family member and be prepared to give time for reactions of fear, guilt, hostility, anger, denial, and even a cathartic response of nonacceptance. *(Engagement 7.8)*

The mother continues to cry uncontrollably.

Mother of the Victim
"How could this be? I saw him this morning! He was excited about his new job. I should have been home here with him. How could I have not known that he would do something like this?"

Paramedic
"I'm so sorry. I cannot even begin to imagine what this is like for you." (Silence) "Is there someone else we should contact?"

Display empathy that is the understanding of another's thoughts and feelings and communicate understanding to them. *(Engagement 7.6)*

The mother shakes her head.

Mother of the Victim
"What's going to happen to him now?"

Paramedic
"I will stay with you as long as I can. My colleague called the hospital while we were talking. We will call the medical examiner's office and arrange transport for your son. The police will be here shortly to stay with you until the medical examiner makes a decision regarding where your son will be taken."

Provide specific information about the disposition of the body with the address and phone number of the agency that will be receiving the body and the time frame in which such disposition will most likely occur. *(Prehospital 25-26)*

SCENARIO ONE FOR ROLE PLAY OR BOALEAN THEATER FORUM FOR EMERGENCY DEPARTMENT NURSES AND PHYSICIANS

Contacting a family member via telephone from the emergency department that a family member has just been brought to the emergency department in critical condition following a stabbing

You are finishing up with a trauma resuscitation that was unsuccessful. A 19-year-old male was stabbed in the left neck and presented with pulsatile bleeding and an expanding hematoma. By the time an airway attempt was made, the cords were not visible. A surgical airway was attempted but severely hindered by the anatomical distortion from the hematoma. The patient did not survive.

The emergency department social worker informs you that she has tracked down the boy's parents. They live in another state, a significant distance from your hospital and their son was attending a local university. You are now faced with breaking news of his death over the phone.

Know the name of the patient, extent of the injuries, and the circumstances of the traumatic event before calling the family. *(Emergency Department 1.2)*

You find a conference room and close the door and after getting settled place a call to the number the social worker gave you.

Conduct the conversation in a quiet private area to reduce any interruptions. *(Emergency Department 1.3)*

After a few rings, a woman answers.

Mother
"Hello."

Physician
"Hello. I need to speak to the parents of William Roberts."

Determine if the contact person is the most appropriate family member, e.g., parent of the victim. *(Emergency Department 1.5.2)*

Mother
"I am his mother. What's the matter? What has he done?"

Physician
"This is Dr. Smith from Hartford Hospital. I have something disturbing to tell you. Is there someone else there that can sit with you while we talk?"

Determine if the contact person is alone in case the call incapacitates her, so that emergency medical service or police can be notified *(Emergency Department 1.5.2)*

Mother
"My husband is here. We are sitting down. Please tell me our Bill is all right!"

Physician
"I have some disturbing news about your son. I took care of him today in the emergency department. The paramedics brought him in by ambulance. Mrs. Smith your son was badly injured and we have no details as to how it happened, but someone stabbed him. The stab wound was in his neck. It was a very serious injury."

Stop at this point and let this initial information be processed.

Explain the injuries and reason for the death. *(Emergency Department 6.3)*

Listen to the response of the family and be prepared to give time for reactions of fear, guilt, hostility, anger, denial, and even a cathartic response of nonacceptance *(Engagement 7.8)*

Recognize that periods of silence may help families process information. *(Engagement 7.11)*

Physician
"We did everything that we could to save your son's life, but I'm sorry to have to tell you that he died."

Avoid euphemisms, e.g., "passed on." *(Engagement 9.3)*

Physician
"I apologize for telling you this over the phone but I thought it best since you live far away."

There may be exceptions to informing relatives over the telephone of the death of a loved one, e.g., relatives who live out of state or are traveling away from home. *(Emergency Department 1.5.5)*

Mother
"How could this happen? You say he was stabbed in the throat but you are trying now to save his life, right?"

Correct any misconceptions or misinterpretations of information. *(Engagement 7.7)*

Physician
"His injury was actually to his neck area. He was brought to our emergency department via ambulance. When he came to us he was unconscious. He was not breathing. We worked very hard to save him; we stopped the bleeding as best we could and gave him blood and oxygen. We had to insert a breathing tube into his windpipe to help him breathe. By the time we got the tube in, his body had been deprived of oxygen for several minutes. His heart stopped as a result and we could not revive him."

Mother
"So he was alive when he got there?"

Physician
"Yes, he was alive but he was unconscious. He was brought directly to one of our specialized rooms we use for severely injured persons and all the members of the trauma team worked hard to try to save him. He was unconscious and there was no indication that he was in pain. Our team was with him the entire time."

Reinforce that the trauma team is with the patient and that all care is being provided. *(Emergency Department 1.7)*

Inform the family that the patient did not feel pain or suffer especially if the patient was unresponsive or dead on arrival. *(Engagement 9.6.1)*

Mother
"It sounds like you did everything possible. Are you sure he did not suffer? I cannot believe this has happened."

Physician
"I can assure you that your son was not suffering. I cannot begin to understand how devastated you must be."

Relieve family's worry that their loved one is suffering or may have suffered. *(Engagement 9.6)*

Mother
"Is he still there in your hospital?"

Physician
"Yes, he is still here. How long do you think it will take you to get here?"

Mother
"It will take us a couple of hours to get there. We will get a flight as soon as we can."

Physician
"I am going to put the nurse on the phone who helped take care of your son. She will give you directions."

Provide emotional and psychological support of the family through the skills of nurses, social workers, or patient advocates when the patient has died. *(Emergency Department 18)*

Nurse
"Hello Mrs. Roberts, my name is Jane and I have been with your son since he arrived in our emergency department. I am so very sorry that your son has died. Tell me what you're thinking right now so I can help you."

Mother
"We can't believe this. Are you sure there is nothing that you can do to bring him back?"

Nurse
"The doctors did everything, Mrs. Roberts, to try to save your son but the injury he had was a very severe one and although we did all we could to try to revive him, the injury to his neck had caused too much bleeding."

Mother starts to cry uncontrollably.

Nurse
"Mrs. Roberts, could you put your husband on the phone please?"

Father
"Hello, this is Mr. Roberts."

Nurse
"Mr. Roberts, I am Jane a nurse at Hartford Hospital where you son was brought with a very severe injury to his neck. Dr. Smith has just explained to your wife what happened; we were unable to save your son due to extensive bleeding. We tried to revive him, but he died. I know you probably want to come to the hospital so let me give you some directions."

Father
"I can't believe this has happened!"

Nurse
"I understand Mr. Roberts. Would you like to speak with the doctor? He is right here. Can you tell me where you will be coming from?"

Mr. Roberts tells the nurse where they live and how long he thinks it will take them to arrive.

Nurse

"Mr. Roberts, when you arrive at Hartford Hospital, go directly to the emergency department entrance and a security guard will meet you there. There is a special parking area that he will direct you to and then once in the emergency department, the guard will bring you to the nurse in charge who will meet you. Dr. Smith will be here to meet with you also."

Communicate clearly and succinctly which hospital is calling, directions to the hospital if needed, where to park when they arrive, where to go once they arrive, who will meet them, and that the physician will speak with them upon their arrival. *(Emergency Department 1.6)*

It is recommended that a specific parking area be designated for families being called to the emergency department in the event a loved one has been injured. *(Emergency Department 1.6.1)*

Nurse

"Mr. Roberts, this is overwhelming news I know, but is there anything else I can do to help you get to the hospital safely?"

SCENARIO TWO FOR ROLE PLAY OR BOALEAN THEATER FORUM FOR EMERGENCY DEPARTMENT NURSES AND PHYSICIANS

Having a discussion between a nurse and physician regarding family presence in emergency department treatment/resuscitation room

There was a gang-related shooting with three victims in a residential area on a Saturday afternoon. A 15-year-old boy shot in the abdomen is being brought to your emergency department. His father is riding in the ambulance with him. As the trauma resuscitation team assembles and you discuss the resuscitation strategy with the team, one of the emergency department nurses brings up the issue of allowing the father to stay with his son in the trauma resuscitation room.

Consider family presence during the administration of life-saving care on a case by case basis. *(Emergency Department 8)*

Nurse
"I heard that the boy's father is with him in the ambulance and he sounded pretty adamant about not leaving his side. I think we should let him stay with his son in the resuscitation room."

Give special consideration when the victim is a child that is seriously injured. *(Emergency Department 8.1)*

Physician
"Are you crazy? No family ever gets to be in **MY** resuscitation room. I think this is insane, there will be blood everywhere and I don't need some parent watching me over my shoulder. Absolutely not, no way will I allow this."

Recognize that some physicians and other health professionals may not agree with family being present in the resuscitation room. *(Emergency Department 8.6)*

Nurse
"But doctor, the administration of the emergency department has discussed this and now there is a procedure for facilitating family presence for those parents who request to be in the room. I have been briefed on the procedure and know what to assess for in terms of making sure that his father will be able to tolerate being there. I will stay with him."

Construct a plan as to how to address these concerns in advance. *(Emergency Department 8.6.1)*

Physician
"The boy's injury sounds really severe from the information we have. There will be a lot of activity in here. It will be up to you to control him. If he makes any false move or he interferes, out he goes!!!!"

Designate a staff professional as the support person for the family member. *(Emergency Department 8.3)*

Nurse
"I don't mind. I really think that if he gets to see what goes on with his son, it will be helpful. He can also help reassure his son who is probably really scared."

Physician
"Good. Well, let's go over a few things so that this goes smoothly. I want you to meet the father and bring him to that corner over there. It has a good view and is not really in the way of the equipment and people in here."

Offer family presence when the care to the patient will not be interrupted. *(Emergency Department 8.2)*

Nurse
"I will get a sense of his overall mood and if he is agitated. If you don't feel right about letting him watch because he is being uncooperative or threatening, let me know sooner rather than later and I can get security involved if we have to."

Assess the family member for signs of combative behavior, intoxication, or potential threat to the healthcare team. *(Emergency Department 8.21-5)*

"We don't know much about him, or if he's had alcohol to drink. I'll make it clear that we're comfortable with him being in the room but that there are some rules he will have to follow."

Family members must agree to follow the instructions of the support person, stand in a designated spot and not interrupt the treatment, and leave if requested by the support person. *(Emergency Department 8.5)*

Physician
"You've been here for quite a few of these gunshot injuries. I'm counting on you to explain what's going on at each stage of the resuscitation so that he understands why we're doing what we're doing. If you have any trouble with that just let me know"

Prepare the family members with an explanation of what to expect during the resuscitation and a description of the procedures being performed. *(Emergency Department 8.4.1-2)*

Nurse
"Sure thing. I'll do what I can because I know how fast things can go and you can meet with him after to fill in the gaps."

Physician
"Thanks for your help. Alright, here come the paramedics. Everyone please be quiet..."

SCENARIO ONE FOR ROLE PLAY OR BOALEAN THEATER FORUM FOR INTENSIVE CARE UNIT PROFESSIONALS

Talking to a family about focusing goals of care on comfort and less on aggressive/curative/injury-specific care

A 70-year-old male pedestrian was hit by a bus while crossing the street and thrown several feet. He suffered a closed head injury, bilateral thoracic injury with pulmonary contusions, bilateral hemothoraces. and high-grade injuries to his liver and spleen. His thoracic spine, pelvis, and left femur were all fractured. It is now hospital day 15 and his neurological status is dismal; he does not respond to verbal or painful stimuli and has no purposeful movements. He is intubated and on the ventilator for support. He has had a splenectomy, external fixation of his femur and angioembolization of his pelvis. His course was complicated by a catheter-related infection, ventilator-associated pneumonia, and acute respiratory distress syndrome (ARDS). His liver has started to fail. He intermittently requires vasopressors for blood pressure support. For the past 3 days he has not made any urine and laboratory studies suggest worsening renal failure. The nephrology consultant wishes to pursue hemodialysis.

Initiate discussion with surrogates in the event that it is the physician's best medical judgment that the patient has a low likelihood of survival and further curative, aggressive treatment is physiologically futile. *(Intensive Care Unit 12)*

Construct a plan of communication with family members that fosters a team approach. Coordinate how conversations with family members are conducted. *(Intensive Care Unit 4.2)*

Start by stating the goals of the meeting. Then proceed to introductions of everyone in the room. It would be especially important to learn who the new family members are and their relationships to the patient.

Learn the relationships to the patient of the family members to whom you are engaging in conversation. *(Engagement 7.4)*

Attending Physician
"We are meeting today to discuss the course of Steven's care over the last few days and to decide on the direction of our care from here on. I know Steven's wife from our discussions at his bedside, but I have not met you before (directed at a new family member) I am Dr. Davies."

Continue the trauma surgeon's involvement as the main contact with the patient and family to maximize shared decision making. *(Intensive Care Unit 10)*

The attending physician should lead the discussion and hopefully has had significant interaction with the key family members and has established trust with them. Start by assessing what the family knows about the care of their loved one and then ask the physician to fill in the gaps and move on to the current problems.

Attending Physician
"Now that everyone has introduced themselves, let us begin. So we can have a place to start, I would like you (directed at family) to share what your understanding of the situation is."

Daughter
"We know Dad is very sick. He has a machine that's breathing for him and he doesn't really wake up. The nurse told me today that the liver lab numbers look worse and now his kidney labs… the…. oh mama what did that nurse say …. Was it the the creatine? Crea-ti-nin? Yes, that laboratory was high and that he needs kidney dialysis. I really want you to do everything doctor. I know it's very serious but I know he'll get better!"

A patient's family member often picks up trends in laboratory values, ventilator settings, and instrument readings through observations and interaction with intensive care unit staff. Do not be surprised.

Families may become overwhelmed with technical jargon and not comprehend the meaning of certain terms. *(Intensive Care Unit 7.3.3)*

This is a time to educate and correct misconceptions if they exist.

Attending Physician
(addressing family) "I've spoken with you several times since his admission and it sounds as if you have a grasp of his condition. We have continued to treat his injuries and problems, but as of today I feel that things are much worse. He already has the ventilator breathing for him, a lung infection and a bloodstream infection. I think that now with his kidneys failing in addition to his liver failure, he will not get better. The problem now is that most of his major body organs are failing."

Initiate discussion with surrogates in the event that it is the physician's best medical judgment that the patient has a low likelihood for survival and further curative, aggressive treatment is physiologically futile. *(Intensive Care Unit 12)*

Wife
"I don't understand doctor, what are you trying to say? Do you think my husband is going to die? I want you to do everything you can to be sure that he survives this. My husband has always been a strong fighter, and I think he can pull through this."

Attending Physician
"Yes, I do think that your husband will not survive this accident. All his body systems are failing and when that happens, it means that the injuries were too severe to survive. You, your family, and I and the others on the team will work this out together. It would help if we knew what your husband might want done if he knew he were in this situation."

Determine the goals of care through a shared decision making model that sees the family and healthcare team as both having input into decisions regarding treatment. *(Intensive Care Unit 11.1)*

Determine options for care based on an assessment of biological objective data, e.g., diagnostic laboratory determinations, physiological measurements, and effectiveness of treatment in conjunction with subjective values and overall expectations of benefit determined by patient and/or family surrogates and burdens such options may incur. *(Intensive Care Unit 15)*

Invite a caregiver that the family trusts to be present at all meetings. *(Intensive Care Unit 20)*

Wife to the Nurse
"Sally, what do you think? You have been so wonderful to my husband and I trust what you think."

Nurse
"I agree with Dr. Davies and another important thing is that he has not really woken up in 15 days. You have been with me when we try to get him to talk. We'll talk to him and move his arms and legs for him but he doesn't really respond."

Daughter
"I don't know. I feel there are times when I think he does feel that we are in the room and that makes me think he is getting better. My mother and I talk to him whenever we can and we always pray for him to get better." (pause)

Attending Physician
"And I think that is good to do. But you need to understand that he has had a severe head injury and it is my opinion that this is the condition he will be in permanently; unable to speak, unable to move, and unable to relate to you. I do not think we can improve his present condition with anything that we can do."

Avoid conveying unrealistic expectations of survival. *(Intensive Care Unit 17.3.2)*

Facilitate the decision process by offering a recommendation. *(Ethics 17.3)*

Wife
"Are you saying he's going to die soon, doctor?"

Attending Physician
"I predict he will die but I can't say exactly when. I can say that when patients are very sick like your husband with similar injuries, infections and organ failure they usually die despite the best medical efforts."

Reinforce the reality of the likelihood of death as needed. *(Intensive Care Unit 17.3.1)*

Daughter
"Isn't the dialysis going to help? And he's on all those medications. Antibiotics? I want you to do everything!!"

Attending Physician
"We have done everything we can. I believe that the dialysis will give him a few more days, but I think he will die even if we try it. I am also concerned that the hemodialysis treatment will be hard for your husband to tolerate and if he cannot tolerate it, for example, if his blood pressure drops, then we cannot continue the treatment since it is causing him more harm than benefit.

Offer only those interventions or treatments that achieve the established goal of care. *(Intensive Care Unit 16)*

Daughter
"Oh no, I can't take this! You have to try, I cannot be without my father. He is supposed to walk me down the aisle when I get married. I just cannot lose him."

Help the family separate the patient's suffering from their suffering. *(Intensive Care Unit 23)*

Attending Physician
"I think it is important to also think of what Mr. West would want in this situation. He did not have a living will or advanced directive. Did he ever talk to you (addressing family) about what he would want to happen if he were ever this sick? What would he think about having a breathing machine and a dialysis machine for the rest of his life?"

Shift the conversation to the patient's best interests and concerns. *(Intensive Care Unit 23.2)*

Wife
"He's always been a fighter. But he's always liked to stand on his own and not rely on anyone. He doesn't like artificial things."

Daughter
"I agree. Remember when he broke his leg and didn't want crutches?"
"Are you saying that we should give up?"

Attending Physician
"Absolutely not. While I don't think that new treatments, like dialysis, are going to make him better, we will always continue measures to make him comfortable. We will not be adding any new treatments. In the event that his heart stops, we can take that as our sign that he is ready to die. I do not recommend any heroic measures such as chest compressions or electric shocks."

Do not use CPR for those patients for whom scientific and empirical evidence has proven that it is not medically indicated, will offer no benefit, and is not indicated based on medical standards of care and is therefore considered physiologically futile. *(Intensive Care Unit 16.1)*

Wife
"What about the breathing tube? I can't bear to think that you are going to pull the plug."

Attending Physician
"I expect that his condition will steadily worsen. It could take a few hours or a few days, that is hard to determine. If we remove the breathing tube, he will die quickly. We would continue to keep him comfortable. I think we have made some significant decisions today. We can see how he does and readdress what to do with the breathing tube tomorrow. Is there other family that we should wait for?"

Avoid the perception that a patient will not receive expert attentive care when the focus is palliation. *(Engagement 11.2)*

Daughter
"I think we should wait for his brother to get here so he can see him."

Waiting for other family members for an extended period of time may put undue stress on those family members who are present. *(Intensive Care Unit 30.1)*

Nurse
"I think that would be good. I'm around all day so we can talk some more about the breathing tube or other questions that you may have."

Social Worker
"And I can arrange a meeting around the same time tomorrow, if his brother can make it."

Attending Physician
"So I think we have agreed that we are not going to proceed with dialysis and that we are not going to perform chest compressions or give him shocks if his heart stops."

Wife
"Yes, now that you have explained it to me, I think it would be too much to put him through dialysis. We want him to be comfortable."

Pastor
"You have made some difficult decisions today. Would you like to meet in Mr. West's room after we leave here and say a prayer with me?"

Assess for needs of the patient and/or family as related to spiritual/religious care. *(Engagement 18)*

SCENARIO TWO FOR ROLE PLAY OR BOALEAN THEATER FORUM FOR INTENSIVE CARE UNIT PROFESSIONALS

Discussing medical futility with a patient's family.

The trauma attending physician, intensive care nurse, and social worker on call meet with the patient's mother to discuss her son. She is accompanied by other siblings and she only speaks Spanish. The siblings speak both Spanish and English.

A 24-year-old **Latino** male was stabbed multiple times in the chest and abdomen and had a delayed transfer from the field due to ongoing violence in the area. He arrived at the trauma center, unconscious with a weak pulse. The patient within minutes of arrival sustained a cardiac arrest. An emergency department thoracotomy, repair of a stab wound to the right ventricle, aortic clamping, and internal cardiac massage were performed. A heart rhythm was restored and the patient was taken to the operating room.

He arrives in the intensive care unit after having a laparotomy that included repairing an injury to the inferior vena cava and a right nephrectomy. Over the next few days he develops hepatic failure, renal failure, and acute respiratory distress syndrome (ARDS). He was started on hemodialysis. Cerebral ischemia is suspected and it is later confirmed by a CT scan that there is no differentiation between gray and white matter and there are other significant signs of acute ischemic damage. The patient has no responses to verbal or painful stimuli and has no demonstration of any purposeful movements.

Trauma Attending Surgeon
"We are meeting to discuss your son's condition. As you know, he was stabbed in the chest and in the abdomen. We repaired a stab wound to his heart and the stab to his abdomen cut a major vessel and severely injured his right kidney. We had to take out his kidney and fix the blood vessel."

Initiate discussion with surrogates in the event that aggressive treatment is physiologically futile. *(Intensive Care Unit 12)*

After appropriate introductions, the purpose of the meeting is stated clearly and the current situation is outlined to the patient's family. A healthcare Spanish-speaking interpreter is summoned to act as translator.

Pause to let these major injuries be processed in the minds of the family.

Trauma Attending Surgeon
"Since then he has done poorly. This is not unexpected due to the severity of his injuries and the delay in time it took to get him to this hospital. His lung, kidneys, and liver are failing. He cannot breathe on his own nor is his kidney working; machines are being used to act as lungs and kidneys. He is also not waking up. His brain was deprived of oxygen for too long before he got to the hospital and I do not think he will regain any function of his brain."

Mother
"Why would his brain not be working, he was stabbed in the chest, right? Is he going to die doctor?"

Trauma Attending Surgeon
"There was not enough blood going to his brain so it shut down. His major organs are failing as a consequence, that is, his liver and his kidney cannot do what they are supposed to do. I think he is going to die within the next day or two. I can tell you that he is not suffering because he cannot feel pain right now and he is unconscious."

Avoid phrases like "meaningful recovery" when discussing imminent death. *(Engagement 9.2)*

Mother
"Isn't there an operation we can do? Maybe a transplant to get him some new organs?"

Determine the medical futility of a treatment by balancing effectiveness, benefits, and burdens. *(Ethics 22)*

Trauma Attending Surgeon
"I am so sorry Mrs. Ruiz, even an organ transplant cannot help your son now. We did everything that we could do to save him and I am so sorry that no more can be done; he almost died on Tremont Street where he was stabbed. There is a machine that is breathing for him right now. He cannot breathe on his own because his lungs have failed. If we take away the breathing machine, his heart will also stop because it will not get oxygen. We have already tried to help his remaining kidney with an artificial kidney machine but that is getting more difficult to do because your son cannot really tolerate being on the machine and his blood pressure drops so we are not able to get the maximum effectiveness of the dialysis treatment."

Offer and describe appropriate and medically indicated options of care based on the patient's condition. *(Intensive Care Unit 13)*

"Right now we are taking an aggressive approach by doing everything that we can to keep your son alive, but it is not going to work. I believe the better solution is to scale back things and focus on keeping him comfortable in the short time that he has left."

Determine options for care based on an assessment of objective data, effectiveness of treatment in conjunction with subjective values, and overall expectations of benefit. *(Intensive Care Unit 15)*

Mother
"Are you saying we should do nothing, doctor?"

Correct the misperception that a patient will not receive expert attentive care when the focus is palliation. *(Engagement 11.3.2)*

Trauma Attending Surgeon
"No, what I am staying is that these heroic measures like the breathing machine and the kidney machine cannot revive your son and make him better, they can only support very basic bodily functions but cannot heal him. We will continue to keep him comfortable with medications as needed. If his heart stops, that is the point in time to say, let him go, let him be in peace and I do not recommend that we do anything to start his heart up like compressions or electrical shocks to his heart if it stops. I also recommend that this be the last dialysis treatment that he has."

Avoid using phrases such as "What do you want us to do?" that minimize the shared decision-making process. *(Intensive Care Unit 17.2)*

Mother
"I want everything to be done, doctor. He's a young man. He is not going to die now. He cannot die now. I need my son—I have no husband and my son supports me and I support him. I want him to have dialysis and all the treatments. You are not God, you cannot decide whether my son lives or dies, that should be in God's hands and right now he is alive and I want you to keep him alive until God decides to take him away."

Trauma Attending Surgeon
"I know how much your son must mean to you Mrs. Ruiz. But this is about his very devastating injuries that have affected his brain."

Help the family or surrogate to separate the patient's suffering from their suffering. *(Intensive Care Unit 23)*

In the event that family members demand care that the physician deems medically futile, the physician should discuss his/her judgments with those who are making decisions for the patient. *(Intensive Care Unit 18.1)*

Trauma Attending Surgeon
"I cannot imagine what you must be going through. If he had a single major injury, I could see him recovering. However, his body as a whole is failing as a result of the injuries he suffered and there is nothing medically we can do to save him. I want to use our efforts to keep him comfortable in his final hours with us."

Mother
"Listen, I go to church every Sunday and I am an active member in my church's community. I believe that God will hear my prayers and save my son. Just you wait and see."

In the event that the family member continues to demand care that is deemed medically futile, obtain a second opinion. *(Intensive Care Unit 18.2)*

Trauma Attending Surgeon
"It is important to pray for your son to not suffer. We will do all that we can to make him comfortable. At this point, we will continue all our current treatments. I will ask that Dr. Carter evaluate your son and speak to you as well. He is the head of our intensive care unit and I think it is important that you hear a second opinion"

In the event that the second medical opinion concurs with the first opinion and the family member still demands futile care, obtain an ethics consultation. *(Intensive Care Unit 18.3)*

APPENDIX 2
SUGGESTED TOPICS FOR PUBLIC DISCOURSE AND DIALOGUE

BRAIN DEATH DEFINITION
(Is it culturally sensitive?)

FUNDING OF MEDICAL CARE FOR THOSE IN A PERSISTENT VEGETATIVE STATE
(Who should pay?)

ADMISSION AND DISCHARGE CRITERIA FOR USE OF INTENSIVE CARE UNITS
(Are they justifiable and are they respected?)

ORGAN DONATION REGISTRY
(Is it universally accepted?)

DNR BRACELETS ON PREHOSPITAL TRAUMA VICTIMS
(Do they matter in trauma scenarios?)

ADVANCE DIRECTIVES FOR PERSONS SUSTAINING TRAUMA
(Are they applicable in trauma scenarios?)

CONTINUATION OF LIFE-SUSTAINING TREATMENTS WHEN THERE IS NO HOPE OF RECOVERY
(Who gets to decide to withdraw such care based on what criteria?)

COST ISSUES ASSOCIATED WITH PROLONGING LIFE THROUGH LIFE-SUSTAINING TREATMENTS
(Can society continue to financially support such care when there is no hope of recovery?)

RESPONSIBILITY FOR CARE OF PATIENTS IN PERSISTENT VEGETATIVE STATE
(Who decides when it may be a burden to family and/or society?)

DISPOSITION OF BODIES FROM SCENE THAT ARE NOT BEING TRANSPORTED TO A HOSPITAL
(Where should they go? What counseling should be available to families?)

FUTILITY DECISION MAKING
(Who decides based on what criteria?)

LIVING WILLS
(Ought mature competent minors have them?)

APPENDIX 3

STATE OF CONNECTICUT
DEPARTMENT OF PUBLIC HEALTH

October 13, 2009

GUIDELINES FOR MRT, EMT - B, I, and PARAMEDIC

DETERMINATION OF DEATH/DISCONTINUATION OF PRE-HOSPITAL RESUSCITATION FOR ADULTS AGE 18 AND OVER NON-MASS CASUALTY SITUATIONS

PROCEDURE FOR DETERMINATION OF DEATH

Local emergency responders and EMS personnel in Connecticut who are trained in any of the National Standard curricula are instructed to follow the most recent national guidelines of the American Heart Association.

All clinically dead patients will receive all available resuscitative measures including cardiopulmonary resuscitation (CPR) unless contraindicated by one of the exceptions defined below. A clinically dead patient is defined as any unresponsive patient found without respirations and without a palpable carotid pulse.

The person who has the highest level of currently valid EMS certification (above MRT level), has active medical control, has direct voice communication for medical orders, and who is affiliated with an EMS organization present at the scene will be responsible for, and have the authority to direct, resuscitative activities.

In the event there is a personal physician present at the scene who has an ongoing relationship with the patient, that physician may decide if resuscitation is to be initiated. In the event there is a registered nurse from a home health care or hospice agency present at the scene who has an ongoing relationship with the patient, and who is operating under orders from the patient's private physician, that nurse (authorized nurse) may decide if resuscitation is to be initiated. If the physician or nurse decides resuscitation is to be initiated, usual medical direction procedures will be followed.

Resuscitation must be started on all patients who are found apneic and pulseless UNLESS the following conditions exist ***(SECTION I (a-d) are applicable to a MRT level provider):***

I. **Traumatic injury or body condition** clearly indicating biological death (irreversible brain death), limited to:

- a. Decapitation: the complete severing of the head from the remainder of the patient's body.
- b. Decomposition or putrefaction: the skin is bloated or ruptured, with or without soft tissue sloughed off. The presence of at least one of these signs indicated death occurred at least 24 hours previously.
- c. Transection of the torso: the body is completely cut across below the shoulders and above the hips through all major organs and vessels. The spinal column mayor may not be severed.
- d. Incineration: 90% of body surface area 3° burn as exhibited by ash rather than clothing and complete absence of body hair with charred skin.

Section (e) and (f) require additional assessment and/or confirmation found under "General Procedures," a-d.

- e. Dependent lividity with rigor mortis (when clothing is removed there is a clear demarcation of pooled blood within the body, and the body is generally rigid). **DOES NOT APPLY TO VICTIMS OF LIGHTNING STRIKES, DROWNING OR HYPOTHERMIA in which case follow your specific protocols.**
- f. Injuries incompatible with life (such as massive crush injury, complete exsanguination, severe displacement of brain matter)

II. Pronouncement of death at the scene by a licensed Connecticut physician or authorized registered nurse.

III. A valid DNR bracelet is present (per CGS 19a-580d), when it:

- a. Conforms to the state specifications for color and construction.
- b. Is intact: it has not been cut, broken or shows signs of being repaired.
- c. Is on the wrist or ankle.
- d. Displays the patient's name and the physician's name.

GENERAL PROCEDURES:

In cases of dependent lividity **with** rigor mortis and in cases of injuries incompatible with life, the condition of clinical death must be confirmed by observation of the following:

a. Reposition the airway and look, listen, and feel for at least 30 seconds for spontaneous respirations; respiration is absent.

b. Palpate the carotid pulse for at least 30 seconds; pulse is absent.

c. Examine the pupils of both eyes with a light; both pupils are nonreactive.

d. Absence of a shockable rhythm with an AED for 30 seconds or lack of cardiac activity with a cardiac monitor [paramedic] (in at least 2 leads) for 30 seconds.

If all the components above are confirmed, no CPR is required.

If CPR has been initiated but all the components above have been subsequently confirmed, CPR may be discontinued and medical direction contacted as needed.

Special Consideration: For scene safety and/or family wishes, provider may decide to implement CPR even if all the criteria for death are met.

If any of the findings are different than those described above, clinical death is NOT confirmed and resuscitative measures must be immediately initiated or continued and the patient transported to a receiving hospital unless paramedic intercept is pending. Termination of resuscitative efforts could then be implemented by the protocol below.

DO NOT RESUSCITATE (DNR) WITH SIGNS OF LIFE

If there is a DNR bracelet or DNR transfer form and there are signs of life (pulse and respiration), EMS providers should provide standard appropriate treatment under existing protocols matching the patient's condition. To request permission to withhold treatment under these conditions for any reason, contact Direct Medical Oversight (DMO).

If there is documentation of a DO NOT INTUBATE (DNI) advanced directive, the patient should receive full treatment per protocols with the exception of intubation. If for any reason intubation is being considered in a patient with a documented DNI directive, DMO must be contacted.

TERMINATION OF RESUSCITATIVE EFFORTS (PARAMEDIC LEVEL ONLY):

NONTRAUMATIC CARDIAC ARREST

Discontinuation of CPR and ALS intervention may be implemented after contact with medical direction if all of the following criteria have been met.

1. Patient must be least 18 years of age.
2. Patient is in cardiac arrest at the time of arrival of advanced life support, no pulse, no respirations, and no heart sounds.
3. ACLS is administered for at least twenty (20) minutes, according to AHA/ACLS Guidelines.
4. There is no return of spontaneous pulse and no evidence of neurological function (non-reactive pupils, no response to pain, no spontaneous movement).
5. Patient is asystolic in two (2) leads.
6. No evidence or suspicion of any of the following: drug/toxin overdose, hypothermia, active internal bleeding, preceding trauma.
7. All Paramedic personnel involved in the patient's care agree that discontinuation of the resuscitation is appropriate.

All seven items must be clearly documented in the EMS patient care report (PCR).

DMO should be established prior to termination of resuscitation in the field. The final decision to terminate resuscitative efforts should be a consensus between the on-scene paramedic and the DMO physician. **CONTACT DMO** for confirmation of terminating resuscitation efforts.

If any of the above criteria are not met and there are special circumstances whereby discontinuation of pre-hospital resuscitation is desired, contact DMO.

Logistical factors should be considered, such as collapse in a public place, family wishes, and safety of the crew and public.

Examples: Inability to extricate the patient, significant physical environmental barriers unified family wishes with presence of a living will.

All patients who are found in ventricular fibrillation or whose rhythm changes to ventricular fibrillation should in general have full resuscitation continued and transported. Patients who arrest after arrival of EMS should be transported.

TRAUMATIC CARDIAC ARREST:

1. Patients must be at least 18 years of age.
2. Resuscitation efforts may be terminated with approval of DMO in any blunt trauma patient who, based on thorough primary assessment, is found apneic, pulseless, and asystolic on ECG upon arrival of emergency medical services at the scene.
3. Victims of penetrating trauma found apneic and pulseless by EMS, should be rapidly assessed for the presence of other signs of life, such as pupillary reflexes, spontaneous movement, response to pain and electrical activity on ECG. Resuscitation may be terminated with permission of DMO if these signs of life are absent. If resuscitation is not terminated, transport per protocol.
4. Do not delay initiating proper BLS resuscitation in order to contact DMO.
5. Cardiopulmonary arrest patients in whom mechanism of injury does not correlate with clinical condition, suggesting a non-traumatic cause of arrest, should have standard ALS resuscitation initiated.

DISPOSITION OF REMAINS:

I. Disposition of dead bodies is not the responsibility of EMS personnel but efforts must be taken to insure that there is a proper transfer of the responsibility for scene security. However, to be helpful to family, police, and others, EMS personnel may assist those who are responsible.

II. When a decision has been made to withhold or withdraw resuscitation, the body may be removed in one of the following ways:

   a. The Office of the Chief Medical Examiner (860-679-3980 or 1-800-842-8820) must be notified of any death, which may be subject to investigation, by the Chief Medical Examiner (CGS19a-407), which includes all deaths that occur outside a health care institution. Normally the police make this notification otherwise EMS personnel should make the notification and document on the patient care record.

   b. If the body is in a secure environment (protected from view by the public or from being disturbed or moved by unauthorized people), the police should be contacted if not present already. The personal physician or coverage must be notified if at all possible and EMS personnel may leave when the patient has been turned over to the police. Example: a death at home

c. If the body is not in a secure environment notify the police. The police may contact the Office of the Chief Medical Examiner for authorization to move the body by hearse, or the medical Examiner may elect to send a vehicle for the body. EMS personnel may leave after turning the scene over to other appropriate authority. Example: death occurring on the street.

d. If the body is not in a secure environment and police have not yet arrived, transport the body to the hospital if scene safety is a concern. Example: death in the street with an unruly crowd of people.

DETERMINATION OF DEATH/DISCONTINUATION OF RESUSCITATION NOTES:

Consider the needs of survivors when considering the discontinuation of resuscitation, especially if crisis management services may be needed. Transport from the scene may be the better option.

Scene management and safety of the crew and public may prevent withholding/discontinuation of resuscitation. In general, do not cease resuscitation in public places/establishments.

Tubes and IV lines may be removed if patient is being picked up by a funeral home. If the patient is deemed a medical examiner's case, leave tubes and lines in place. In all cases of trauma, tubes and IV lines must be left in place.

Documentation of all encounters with the patient's family, personal physician, scene physician or nurse, medical examiner, law enforcement, and DMO should be on the PCR.

DNR TRANSFER FORM

a. To transmit a DNR order during transport by an EMS provider between healthcare institutions, the DNR order shall be documented on the DNR transfer form.

b. The DNR transfer form shall be signed by a licensed physician or a registered nurse and shall be recognized as such and followed by EMS providers.

c. The DNR remains in place during transport as well as to the point of admission to the receiving facility.

REVOCATION OF THE DNR

The patient's representative, according to Connecticut statutes, cannot revoke a valid DNR order.

However, in the event that EMS providers cannot verify the DNR status, the patient should be transported with normal care protocols followed.

A copy of all PCRs documenting pre-hospital deaths must be provided to medical direction within 24 hours of the event.

APPENDIX 4

Department of Public Health **Public Health Code**

DNR Orders

19a-580d-1. Definitions

As used in sections 19a-580d-1 through 19a-580d-9 of the Regulations of Connecticut State Agencies:

(1) "Attending physician" means the Connecticut licensed physician selected by or assigned to a patient, who has primary responsibility for the treatment and care of the patient. Where more than one physician shares such responsibility, any such physician may act as the attending physician.

(2) "Authorized representative" means a person who is otherwise authorized by law to provide consent to the issuance or revocation of a DNR order for an incapable or incompetent patient.

(3) "Department" means the Connecticut Department of Public Health.

(4) "Designated agency" means either a healthcare institution or a physician licensed by the department.

(5) "Do Not Resuscitate order" or "DNR order" means an order written by a Connecticut licensed physician to withhold cardiopulmonary resuscitation, including chest compressions, defibrillation, or breathing or ventilation by any assistive or mechanical means including, but not limited to, mouth-to-mouth, mouth-to-mask, bag-valve mask, endotracheal tube, or ventilator for a particular patient.

(6) "DNR bracelet" means the bracelet approved by the department for the transmission of a `Do Not Resuscitate' order and meeting the requirements of section 19a-580d-4.

(7) "DNR transfer form" means a form approved by the department for the transmission of a `Do Not Resuscitate' order issued by a licensed physician.

(8) "Emergency Medical Services provider" or "EMS Provider" means a person, association, or organization who provides immediate or life saving transportation and medical care away from a hospital to a victim of sudden illness or injury, and who may also provide invalid coach services.

(9) "Healthcare institution" means an institution licensed or regulated under chapter 368v of the Connecticut General Statutes.

(10) "Medical direction" means the provision of medical advice, consultation, instruction and authorization to appropriately trained or certified personnel by designated staff members at sponsor hospitals.

(Effective December 30, 1996.)

19a-580d-2. DNR transfer form

(a) To transmit a DNR order between healthcare institutions or during transport by an EMS provider between healthcare institutions, the DNR order shall be documented on the DNR transfer form.

(b) The DNR transfer form signed by a licensed physician or a registered nurse shall be recognized as such and followed by healthcare institutions and EMS providers.
(Effective December 30, 1996.)

19a-580d-3. Transfer and recognition of DNR orders when patients are transported

(a) When a patient who is to be transferred between healthcare institutions has a DNR order which is to remain in effect during and after the transfer, that order shall be documented on a DNR transfer form which is signed by the physician who entered the DNR order or by a registered nurse who attests to the existence of such order. The DNR transfer form or a legible copy shall be sent with the patient when the patient is transferred to another healthcare institution.

(b) The DNR transfer form or a legible copy shall be retained with the patient's medical record.

(c) The DNR transfer form or a legible copy or a DNR bracelet shall be shown to all EMS providers by the healthcare facility staff person who transfers care of the patient to the EMS providers. The EMS provider shall show the DNR transfer form or a legible copy or a DNR bracelet to a nurse or physician at the receiving healthcare institution or, in the absence of a nurse or physician, the person in charge of patient care.

(d) Any healthcare institution receiving a patient with a DNR transfer form, a legible copy, or DNR bracelet shall honor the DNR order until such time as admitting orders are written in accordance with the healthcare institution's policies.

(e) When a patient has a DNR order which is to remain in effect after discharge from a healthcare institution to home, that patient shall be offered a DNR bracelet by the healthcare institution prior to discharge.

(f) Any EMS provider receiving a patient with a DNR transfer form or a legible copy or a DNR bracelet shall honor the DNR order.
(Effective December 30, 1996.)

19a-580d-4. DNR bracelets

(a) A DNR bracelet shall be the only valid indication recognized by EMS providers that a DNR order exists for patients outside a healthcare institution, other than those patients received by an EMS provider directly from a healthcare institution. A valid DNR bracelet shall:
   (1) be of a design approved by the department,
   (2) be affixed to the patient's wrist or ankle,
   (3) display the patient's name and attending physician's name, and
   (4) not have been cut or broken at any time.

(b) A DNR bracelet shall be recognized and honored by healthcare institutions and EMS providers.

(c) A patient or the patient's authorized representative may obtain a DNR bracelet from any designated agency based on a written order from the patient's attending physician.
   (1) The designated agency shall maintain a permanent record including a copy of the written DNR order.
   (2) A designated agency may obtain DNR bracelets and DNR transfer forms from the organization selected by the department to maintain a central supply of such items.

(Effective December 30, 1996.)

19a-580d-5. EMS providers

DNR patients under the care of EMS providers shall be given medical care as determined by consultation with medical direction, recognizing the limitations of the DNR order.
(Effective December 30, 1996.)

19a-580d-6. Assistance by attending physicians

When requested by a patient or his authorized representative the attending physician who issued the DNR order shall:

(a) provide the patient with information on how to contact a designated agency, or

(b) if a patient is unable to obtain a DNR bracelet from any other source, the attending physician shall obtain and provide one.
(Effective December 30, 1996.)

19a-580d-7. Revocation

A DNR order may be revoked by the patient or authorized representative in any of the following ways:

(a) Removing the bracelet from the patient's extremity, or

(b) telling an individual licensed healthcare provider or certified emergency medical technician. Such healthcare provider or emergency medical technician shall enter, or cause to be entered, the contents of the statement in the patient's permanent medical record and notify the attending physician and the physician who issued the DNR order.

(Effective December 30, 1996.)

19a-580d-8. Provision for patients with certain considerations

(a) Nothing in these regulations shall be construed to limit the authority of the commissioner of mental retardation under subsection (g) of section 17a-238 of the general statutes concerning orders applied to persons receiving services under the direction of the commissioner of mental retardation.

(Effective December 30, 1996.)

19a-580d-9. Ethical, philosophical, religious objections

(a) Healthcare providers who have an ethical or philosophical, or religious objection to implementing a DNR order shall turn over care of the patient without delay to another provider who will implement the DNR order. Pending the assumption of care by another provider, the DNR order shall be followed.

(Effective December 30, 1996.)

APPENDIX 5

STATE OF CONNECTICUT

DEPARTMENT OF MENTAL RETARDATION

End-of-Life Decisions

Policy No. I.E.PO.007
Issue Date: May 26, 2004
Subject: End-of-Life Decisions Effective Date: upon release **Section**: Health and Safety

A. Policy Statement

The Department of Mental Retardation recognizes the rights of individuals to make decisions about their health care including end-of-life decisions as do all Connecticut citizens. End-of-life decisions include: advance directives, do not resuscitate orders and withholding and/or withdrawing life support.

Individuals' rights to make end-of -life decisions were delineated in the 1990 Federal Self-Determination Act and implemented in Connecticut in a December 1, 1991 memorandum from Connecticut's Attorney General (see attached). This act defined patient's rights to make decisions about their health care and their right to formulate advance directives. The act also mandated health facilities to develop written policies on how to implement such patient rights, and ruled that the provision of care must not be conditioned on the formulation of advance directives, including Do Not Resuscitate (DNR) orders.

Advance directives are prepared before any condition occurs which prevents the person's participation in decision-making. Advanced directives recognized in Connecticut are:

1. Living Wills
2. Health Care Agent
3. Durable Power of Attorney for Health Care Decisions

The process and applicability of *advance directives* for individuals served by the department are delineated in DMR Procedure I.D.PR.007a, Advance Directives.

A Do Not Resuscitate (DNR) order may be instituted to withhold cardiopulmonary resuscitation after respiration and cardiac function have ceased, as a natural progression of the dying process. A DNR order may be instituted for an individual who is terminally ill when the physician has determined that:

1. resuscitation would be of no benefit because the natural course of the individual's medical condition would result imminently in death
2. the institution of resuscitative measures, if successful, would only postpone the moment of death for a brief period and
3. resuscitation would not be in the best interest of the individual.

A "do not resuscitate" order may be compatible with maximal therapeutic efforts, short of resuscitation or may be accompanied by further orders that limit or withhold other identified medical interventions. These decisions shall be based on the specific needs of the individual and shall meet the criteria detailed in DMR Procedure No. I.E.PR.007c, Withholding Cardiopulmonary Resuscitation. Decisions to withdraw and/or withhold life support may be appropriate for individuals with a terminal diagnosis. These decisions shall be based on the specific needs of the individual and shall be reviewed by the department as delineated in DMR Procedure No. I.D.PR.007b, Withholding and/or Withdrawing Medical Treatment.

Neither the commissioner nor any employee of the Department of Mental Retardation has the legal authority to give consent for or to rescind a "do not resuscitate" order or any other end-of-life decision for any individual. Consent must be obtained from the individual, individual's family, guardian or conservator of person.

I.E.PO.007 End of Life Decisions 1

The department's role is to assure that neither the individual's retardation nor level of retardation prior to his or her medical difficulty is considered in the decision to issue a "do not resuscitate" order and/or other end-of-life decisions and to otherwise prevent discrimination on the basis of mental retardation in the delivery of medical services and medical decision making.

B. Applicability

This procedure shall apply to all individuals for whom the department bears direct or oversight responsibility for medical care. This includes people living in programs operated, licensed, and/or funded by the department, including non-Connecticut residents living in such facilities. It also applies to people receiving supported living services, receiving respite services in DMR-operated or -funded facilities, and people living in facilities licensed by the Department of Public Health if the department was involved with the placement decision.

This procedure also applies to non-Connecticut residents who receive services in DMR-operated, -funded and/or -licensed facilities or programs.

Staff from public and private sector shall adhere to this policy.

C. References

Statutes

Federal

1990 Federal Self-Determination Act

State

CGS 17a-238, Rights of Persons with Mental Retardation

CGS 19a-469

CGS 19a-575, Living Wills

CGS 19a-576, Health Care Agent

CGS 19a-580 (d), Transfer of DNR Orders

CGS 45a-562, 1-43, 1-5a, Durable Power of Attorney for Health Care Decisions

Rules, Regulations and Policy – External

19a-580d-1, et. Seq., Transfer of DNR Orders

Rules, Regulations and Policy or Instructions – DMR

DMR I.F.PO.001, Abuse and Neglect Prevention

DMR I.F.PR.00, Abuse and Neglect Prevention, Reporting, Notification, Investigation, Resolution and Follow-up

DMR I.E.PR.007a, Advance Directives (Living Wills)

DMR I.E.PR.007b, Withholding or Withdrawing Medical Treatment

DMR I.E.PR.007c, Withholding Cardiopulmonary Resuscitation

Case Management Procedures

Client Rights

I.E.PO.007 End of Life Decisions 2

APPENDIX 6

Interprofessional Team Communication Form

Documenting Discussions with Family/Other Decision Makers

Patient ID Sticker

Date:________________________

Decisional Capacity

☐ Yes ☐ No

If No, reason for loss of capacity to make own healthcare decisions:

____

If No, who is making patient's healthcare decisions:

____

Relationship of above decision maker to patient:

☐ Spouse ☐ Parent ☐ Other: __________________

Advance Directives

☐ No ☐ Yes ☐ Living Will ☐ Healthcare Representative

If Yes, advance directives are in the patient's record:

☐ Yes ☐ No, but have been requested

Code Status

☐ Full Code Status ☐ DNR Order Written Date: ______________________

Code Status discussed with:

☐ Surrogate Decision Maker Date:______________Your Name: ________________________

Others ____

Discussion Regarding Goals of Care, Code Status, or Prognosis

Interprofessional Health Team Members Present:

____

____

____

Family, Surrogate Decision Maker Present, Others Present:

____

____

____

Synopsis of Conversation and Outcome:

____

____

____

____

____

____

____

____

INDEX